Paul ;

Salsa

7. P.m.

Sunny Side

of a
rainy life

Contact Hilford

250· 287·923·0281

BY ELIZABETH MORGAN

DISCLAIMER
To protect the privacy of physicians, their names have been changed and some physical features have been modified.

Produced by:

FriesenPress

Suite 300 – 852 Fort Street
Victoria, BC, Canada V8W 1H8

www.friesenpress.com

Distributed to the trade by The Ingram Book Company

table of contents

dedication

For my valiant husband, Ron Morgan who has stood faithfully with me: daily bearing the burden of my extended illness, guiding our sons, covering us with prayer, cheering me on with his crazy humour and courting me with his unfailing devotion.

~

For our sons, Mark and Paul Morgan who have eased the way with their love, laughter and belief that we could get through this.

~

And most of all... for the One who has led us all the way and deserves honour above all others!

Lord, You have been our dwelling place
throughout all generations.
~Psalm 90:1

disclaimer

To protect the privacy of physicians, their names have been changed and some physical features have been modified.

heartfelt thanks

Adele Wickett for her professional edits and amusing comments about my grammatical errors.

Richard Sherbaniuk for his thorough proofreading, excellent edits, and passionate support.

Ian West for designing a cover that we love! And for his belief in our project.

Colleen McGinnis for working her magic on my book photos.

Jacquie Lambi who urged me to write this book in the first place.

~

Hazel West for inviting me into her select writing group, for mentoring and pushing me to do better.

Karen Gibbs for her loving nudges over the decades, reminding me to keep on writing this book (be faithful to your call, get out that pen again and blow some cobwebs out of the system).

My Mother, Margaret Reimer, who cultivated in me an appreciation for written expression.

My Dad, Alfred Reimer, who gave me a taste for storytelling.

~

All My Caregivers – Renal Doctors, Nurses And Other Specialists – who delivered care with diligence, compassion, a listening ear, and humour.

All Those Generous Souls who offered to be my donor: my siblings, relatives, friends and some of Ron's staff.

All Our Friends And Family who drew alongside us to cheer, support, and pray with us.

~

My Brother, Dave Reimer who gave me the gift of life – the greatest encouragement of all.

prologue

Were you angry with God?

Tonight we go all-out for our company of two — a retired general practitioner and his wife. We light a candle and set out the new cut-glass dinnerware we found at *Value Village*. When Jack and Joan arrive they comment on the coziness of our tiny condo overlooking Victoria's harbour front and the Juan de Fuca Strait.

We don't usually invite company to dinner — sometimes a single person, but we socialize in small doses. I need to conserve my energy and Ron's patience grows thin with small talk.

We joke about how pleased we feel with our "find" at the thrift shop earlier that day. This information likely amuses our guests no end. Ron has even snapped pictures of our table setting to mark the occasion.

Over our comfort meal of shepherd's pie and fresh green beans our guests ask many questions about my health. They wonder how we survived the decade-long misdiagnosis of my illness and the grinding reality of the years that followed.

Joan remarks that now we are visiting amiably with a doctor and we don't seem bitter about the run-around that his profession has given us in the past. "You two seem very happy," she adds.

We admit we still have our moments of frustration with medical carelessness.

They probe further, not intrusively, but with a sincere interest in something they have not experienced. Recently arrived at our sixth decade, Ron and I are still amazed that I have reached this landmark in one piece, more or less – with a few losses, gains and revised body parts.

Jack poses a new question: "Do you think that what you went through made you a better person?" Long pause on our part. No quick answer for that one.

More questions. "Were you angry with God? Bitter? Did your faith in God grow stronger?"

Yes, to all three.

"Marriages often do not survive serious illness," Joan comments. "What brought you through thirty-eight years together?"

Ron and I exchange smiling glances. Now there's a story we like to tell! Our love story fills us with gratitude.

Doctor Jack points out that as a former physician, current sponsor of a seniors' club and a spiritual news writer he has experienced many opportunities to ask his patients and elderly acquaintances how they cope with the unwelcome news of ill health or other misfortune.

"People tell me that there's no point to suffering," says Jack. "They say that nothing good comes from it."

Our guest's last comment mobilizes me. I long to address these heartrending big questions of life — ones I have also entertained when going through the worst of times.

Is there a point to suffering? Can any good come from it? What does God have to do with our struggles? Does He even care?

How to respond to these cries of the heart? I can only tell my story – a story God gave me – one I have been mapping for decades. And so I offer up to readers another way of viewing one's own life and the adversity that comes to all of us.

~

chapter 1
Fire in the sky, itches on the skin, sunshine on the shadow

I can still picture myself as a little girl with brown braids skipping alongside my bigger brothers and parents to the church service down the road from our white frame house. Joining other children who sat on child-sized chairs, I listened to our teacher lead us in songs and stories about Jesus.

"It can't wait," the lady said. "Jesus is returning some day for those who love Him." She showed us where this was written in the Bible. "Do you know if you're ready to meet Him?" she asked.

Oh no, I wasn't sure at all.

As though she guessed my inner response she added, "It's the most important decision a person will ever make... don't wait until it's too late."

Later I had occasion to ponder this challenge from the back seat of my father's 1951 Austin van. My dad steered our car onto the road out of Steinbach while Mom warned my brothers to hold down the racket.

Feet not yet able to reach the floor mat, I sat forward and pressed my face against the cool window. Hydro poles marked off my beloved prairie. The sun began its descent behind a distant barn. Blue sky faded to a curtain of shadows as our car bumped over the gravel road. When I felt the smooth whine of tires I knew we had reached the highway to Winnipeg. Yawning, I settled back into my seat, expecting a long drive before our visit with city cousins.

Our car slowed behind a long row of other vehicles. What was wrong? My brothers commented on the stink of tar being poured and raked by workmen in overalls. I rolled my window down. Pots of fire and wooden barriers guided our vehicles along a winding detour beside the paving site.

How intriguing! The thickening darkness, the sharp odour and the blackened fire pots boded something significant about to happen. As the city skyline rolled into view, the sky exploded with colour. Blazing arcs and starbursts flashed skyward before plummeting back to earth.

Mesmerized, I gripped the back of my mother's seat, my eyes round as full moons.

Was this dark night of fire and light the time predicted in my teacher's Bible? The prospect of glimpsing Jesus thrilled me with both joy and terror. I'd heard stories of Jesus gathering little children around Him. But I also heard stories of Jesus warning people not to depend on their own way to heaven.

I doubted that I was ready to meet Him – and now it was too late.

Noticing my dismay one brother poked me. "What's the matter, Lizzy, haven't you ever seen fireworks before?"

Oh… was that all?

Wrapping thin arms around myself I fell back against the seat. The drama of that night inspired a course of inquiry. Was Jesus really coming back, and would I be ready?

~

Drumming the backboards with bare feet I waited for relief. My eyes traced the cut-out moon at the top of the door. I preferred not to think about the creatures that might be creeping up from the bogs beneath my bottom or lurking in the other shadowy corners of our outhouse. At any moment something with hairy legs might ascend along my foot. Shuddering, I scratched the scabs along my foot, my leg, my torso. Would this itching never end?

I rather enjoyed this quiet time alone in our outhouse below my mother's garden; the place where a girl could escape from her noisy household. I didn't even mind the stink of muck below – as long as I was careful not to inhale, look down or fall in.

Gripping the rough seat more tightly I reached for a sheet of last week's *Carillon News* and tore off one piece, and then another.

"Lizzie, hurry up, you've been in there long enough!" Dale banged on the door.

Finally I unlatched the door. Shoving him with my shoulder I stuck out my tongue as I trundled back up the dirt path to the house. I ran my hands along the Dutch boy and girl lawn ornaments cut out by my father and lovingly detailed by my mother. The evening air carried the scent of her flowers — more inviting than the medicinal smell drifting through the screen door.

A bald light hung from the kitchen ceiling highlighting a metal tub on the painted floorboards where my mother knelt, washing my younger brother with lye soap.

"Come Elizabeth," my mother sighed, "take off your sundress and Kenny, move over." As I squished in beside him, Mom lathered my head and arms. The water felt soothing. My mother's hands looked as thinly worn as her face. She lifted Kenny from the tub and toweled him down, then me.

Her daily tasks not nearly done yet, she called to my three older brothers, born less than three years apart: "Billy, Davey, Dale — come, we haven't got all night!"

The Three Musketeers (my dad's name for them) jostled one another for position as Mom tossed their clothes onto the stack of laundry to be washed later that evening. Mom refilled the pot on the stove.

"How many times do I have to tell you kids? Don't scratch your scabs — you'll only make them worse!" she scolded.

She had to remind us many times a day. Limp strands of brown hair slipped from her headscarf as she knelt to repeat the routine of scrubbing, rinsing, and toweling down each wiggling, itching body.

While we put on our pajamas I heard the sound of clothes being dragged along the washboard, back and forth, back and forth. My mother didn't even bother to whistle or sing her usual happy tune.

Watching my mother's heavy movements, I wondered about the growing mound around her slender waist. And did the wash bucket hold her tears? I wanted to cry too.

Every day that summer, Mom washed and pegged our clothes onto the clothesline, along with our bedding and towels. No time to apply a fresh coat of paint to our kitchen table and chairs or coax delicate designs from her brush across the chair backs.

"Liestje, ('little one') are you still up? Get yourself to bed. Billy, help your sister say her prayers."

I do not recall what my oldest brother and I said to God but I welcomed our comforting evening routine. Surely God was listening and maybe even looking out for us.

All that care-worn summer of '51 we suffered quarantine until our skin condition cleared up.

Before Thanksgiving my mother delivered a good-natured baby sister for us, named Susan Ann. But the strain of nightly baths for five children and the hand-scrubbed laundry had taken their toll on Mom. Another change may have been the last straw.

~

Whenever my father returned from one of his many business trips to the east he liked to treat us to a brick of Neapolitan ice cream, a bundle of bananas or a barrel of crisp Macs from the Niagara orchards. On one particular return he brought us an even bigger surprise.

With glee in his sky-blue eyes he announced that we were moving to another province. His prestigious promotion with a trucking company meant a transfer to their Ontario center. My dad promised us an adventure; he naturally characterized every bend in the road as an adventure. We six would travel with Mom by passenger train from Winnipeg while Dad would drive ahead of us with the furniture and meet us at the train station in Windsor. Some of us met this move with a heavy heart.

For me it meant leaving behind my beloved paternal grandma whose nearby home had provided a welcoming retreat. There I was made to feel like the centre of her universe, even though I was only one of a dozen grandchildren. Grandma invited me to walk together through her garden of chokecherry and crabapple trees and flowers, or to talk with her in the morning while she sat before her dressing table brushing her long brown hair and braiding it into a coil at the nape of her neck.

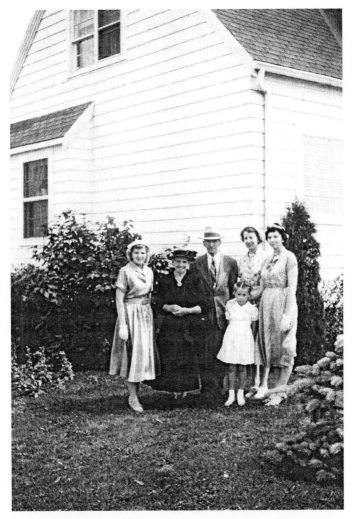

Visiting my Grandma's house, Steinbach 1952

Years later I learned from a cousin that she too believed that Grandma favoured her. This gentle bent woman who suffered severe scoliosis and arthritis, prayed for all her family with quiet determined faith, making each of us feel dearly loved. Even my wary mother said that she had the best mother-in-law in the world.

~

What must this move have meant for my worn-out mother? Like Dad she embraced adventure, but subsequent events exposed a spirit depleted by sorrow and distress.

Mom told me stories about how a part of her was forever bound with her people, her ancestral home — the place where it all began for her. Orphaned as a baby, my mother grew up in her grandfather Jacob's big farmhouse along with her deceased mother's nine brothers and sisters who took turns raising this infant niece as their own. Her youngest Aunt Minna, who became more like a sister, now lived in the cherished homestead. There we spent hours playing while Mom and Dad visited.

I suspect my mother's morale began to tear like a piece of threadbare cloth as our train pulled her away from the family who had nurtured her into adulthood. But she never grieved in front of us. Instead she chose to take hold of joy wherever she could find it.

As was often her habit when carrying heartache, Mom forced a smile. She encouraged us to enjoy the passing scenes, to wave at the farmers pausing in their fields and at the children running to greet us. She urged us to inhale the scent of towering pine trees as we passed along the bluffs and lakes of Northern Ontario.

~

Dad met us at the Windsor station and drove us to our next home, a cottage in touristy Alexander Beach. We stayed here only about a year, long enough to complete our family with the arrival of a seventh baby, James, in 1952.

During our time in cottage country I grew aware of an unyielding sorrow weighing my mother down. Her weeping seeped through closed doors. Did she yearn for her extended family? Her grief plowed my spirit with sympathy: a fierce though silent protectiveness welled up within me. I lingered nearby to absorb her sadness as though this could lessen her isolation and lighten her load — a rather serious task for a six-year-old to undertake.

Apparently another source for her depression during this time concerned my oldest brother Bill, age twelve, who was diagnosed with severe visual loss. The recommendation: a School for the Blind. Billy would eventually leave us to board at a special school in Brantford, Ontario.

The glossy wooden plaque that hung over my mother's bed depicted Jesus kneeling at a rock with pleading eyes raised to heaven, tears falling like blood. Billy's blindness became my mother's Gethsemane. Here, as never before, she identified with this Man of Sorrows; she too had knelt, beseeching Father God to let this cup pass.

Whether she had added, "Yet not my will but Thine," I don't know. But years later she told me God heard her cry and drew alongside to walk this path with a broken-hearted mother.

I'm sure my father also wept within the privacy of his reflections and prayers, processing this in his own way. I'll never know how since he kept these things to himself. Yet it comforted me to watch him reading the Bible he often held on his lap in the evening.

My mom probably found solace in her garden. Often I would join her as she inspected the flowerbeds surrounding our cottage home, rich with patches of fall blooms — asters, mums and marigolds. I smile at how unimpressed I used to be with the pungent odour of these autumn varieties. Today these same sharp smells remind me of my mother's resilience and fierce determination to overcome the hurts of life, to plant and nurture a garden in spite of the inevitable weeds.

Long after my mother's garden succumbed to November frost, the wiggling life growing in her womb warned of James' imminent arrival.

Mom hurried us off to Mrs. Wilson, the neighbour whose back yard touched ours. I recall a warmly cheerful round woman who designed sequined dance and skate costumes for stars like Barbara Ann Scott. On our last day with this kind friend she served us a puzzling brew of white bread scraps floating on a sea of hot milk. Perhaps her creative skills did not extend to the kitchen, or more likely, she was run ragged by our noisy energy. Who else would take on a family of six children with such patience?

When Mrs. Wilson finally ushered us home we found our new brother lying on the living room daybed. Someone snapped a photo of Kenny and me resting our elbows against the bed, our faces a study in wonder at this tiny bundle who waved his arms as though equally happy to meet us.

~

As winter rolled into spring and early summer, we moved to nearby Windsor. We children explored every nook of our new home, a roomy white two-story house with a large yard, trees and an iron fence. My mother especially enjoyed the spreading ash tree shading the front yard and porch.

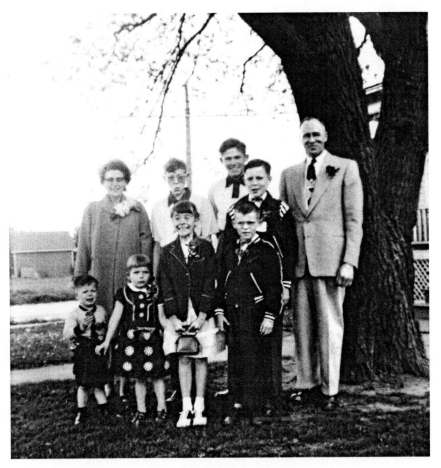

Mom and Dad with their brood of seven, Windsor, Back row: Mom,
Bill, Dave. Dale, Dad, Front Row: James, Susan, me, Ken

This move meant that Dad's company office and trucking warehouse stood on the other side of our fence. We could visit him any
time we wished! Dad relished showing us the clacking *Teletype*
machine as it delivered a continuous scroll of messages, and
the big transports being loaded or unloaded. As manager of the
company's eastern division my dad oversaw the office staff, truck-
ers and shipping. This must have been a dream come true for my
father who had previously trained bus drivers and operated his own
chicken hatchery.

Railway tracks lined the other side of the company yard, a feature that became a bane for our mother trying to keep her brood safe, and for me as I tried to harness James' rambunctious and fearless spirit.

However these same tracks also gave me much pleasure. My father liked to amuse people with stories about his daughter, Elizabeth, who could not fall asleep until the evening train came through. Sounds that interrupted sleep for the others enhanced mine. The blasts of the whistle, the hiss of the locomotive, and the clacking trundle of the wheels evoked the soothing memory of our move by train the previous year, when I developed a love for the rocking motion as we slept in our bunks.

~

With approaching summer my father decided we should all take a road trip to Steinbach, perhaps with the thought of giving my mom's spirits a lift. We rented an upstairs apartment on Main Street, but the stifling heat became unbearable for Mom.

So we retreated to our Aunt Minna's spacious farm, the homestead where our mother grew up. At this warm, fun-loving place we explored the barns and fields all day long with our country cousins.

I wonder if this reunion with my mother's roots held highlights of pure delight for her — or had she turned a corner of no return? Did the combination of oppressive heat, so many active children, the toil of that summer of skin infection, the separation from her home town, and then the burden of Bill's impending move to a School for the Blind set the stage for the next drama? Inevitably she knew that this little bit of bliss with her childhood family would soon end.

~

Exactly why or how it happened I don't know. The scenes melted into one another. One moment we children chased each other among the trees in the farm garden and the next we stood on a long sloping lawn in Winnipeg with Dad, scanning the windows of a red-brick building. My father pointed to a third story window where a slender woman waved. She was our mother. We took turns visiting her in a sitting room. Dad explained that Mom needed a rest and this hospital would provide that.

After our last visit with Mom we once more stood on the hospital lawn looking upward and waving farewell. How I wished it were time to bring Mom home. But school season would begin soon and we needed to return to Windsor.

Mom looked like a caged bird that had forgotten the words to her song. It felt sad to watch her peering at us from her hospital window with bars but our mother needed time to return to health without a litter of children underfoot. A hanky fluttered from behind her window.

The distance between us grew as we drove away in our tiny Austin van heaped high with suitcases. Our mother's receding figure left an indelible mark upon my spirit.

Over time I realized it was my mother's faith in God that helped her withstand this test of separation and physical exhaustion. Someday the melody to her song would return.

~

Meanwhile Dad ensured our trip home to Windsor would be an adventure of sightseeing and roadside picnics with supplies bought from groceterias along the way: cold ham, rolls, pickles, tomatoes and potato salad. Dad enjoyed lining up his children for another snapshot in front of our vehicle with the northern pines of a Canadian highway as our backdrop. The forest green corduroy jumper I wore reminded me of Mom, who had fashioned it for me from an outgrown pair of boy's trousers.

Even service station stops were fun. My father told us to be sure we all made our pit stops while he had the car filled up. "Gas in and gas out," he used to joke at every fill-up. I cringed with embarrassment. Now I smile with appreciation at my dad's ability to look at the lighter side of life. Often he invited us to choose a soft drink for the next leg of the journey. Oh the anticipation of holding the chilled contours of a glass bottle of grape, orange crush or cherry soda in my hands!

Whenever we passed a fleet of Reimer transport trucks my Dad honked and waved. He knew all the truck drivers by name. "There's Curly," Dad would chuckle, "and there's Rolly".

When we finally turned onto the Reimer trucking lot on George Avenue we spilled out, eager to reacquaint ourselves with the home we had moved into only months earlier.

How I wished my mother could have been here to share this experience with us. No one could fill the space meant for her alone. Not my siblings, though they crowded the waning August days with hide and seek games in our yard and exploration of our neighbourhood. Not my cheerful Aunt Jean, wife of Dad's brother John, though she faithfully cooked, cleaned and laundered for us; nor her daughter, Linda, who became my bosom friend during those Windsor years.

~

The opening day of the fall school session — grade one — found me with knees knocking as I stood outside Ada C. Richards School.

Everything overwhelmed me with newness: the school setting, the teacher, my classmates, and the instructions. I fumbled with simple directions for folding a paper into squares. What would the others think? Would they laugh? Would they ignore me at recess? I couldn't let them see my confusion. As I peeked to watch how others were doing each task, someone whispered, "Copycat." Someone else followed the chant. Copycat! This disapproving label raised my anxiety. I believed I could never learn the new tasks and would forever copy others. At night when bad dreams awakened me I cried out for my mother's comfort.

~

Then — oh glorious day — my mother came home!

Life returned to normal. My mom again presided over the kitchen and household affairs, whistling as she applied a fresh coat of yellow paint to kitchen walls and chairs. Enlisting my dad to install French windows in the dining room, Mom ordered ruffled white curtains to adorn her sun-filled nook.

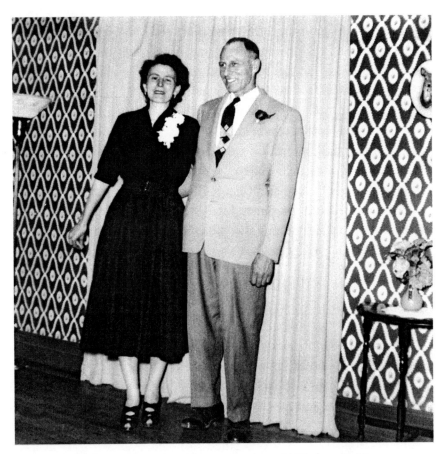

A happy day when Mom comes home! Windsor 1955

Together again, our family joined Campbell Avenue Baptist Church in downtown Windsor where I learned children's choruses and the great classic hymns of my parents' and grandparents' generations. I'm sure that my God-honouring father had already re-established us with church life during my mom's absence. But this memory is connected to her return since Mom added the extra touch to our Sunday finery. She made bonnets along with dainty gloves and purses for Susan and me; and she dealt with that last minute ironing of wrinkled pleats and collars.

As was her habit my mother once again enquired about what we had learned in Sunday School. I showed her the Wordless Book my teacher had given our class members – a book with four glossy coloured pages, each one symbolizing a different but related fact. This tiny treasure played an important role in leading me later to make a critically life-directing decision.

So did my mom's input. Even after Mom's return I continued to have bad dreams. But whenever she heard me cry out she hurried to my bedside and lay beside me. She smelled of her nightly beauty treatment — *Pond's* cold cream — the fragrance of comfort. Mom asked what troubled me and then invited me to ask Jesus to give me good dreams. Cold cream and Jesus got me through many a night of childhood anxiety about the monsters of my daytime hours — trying to keep up with the class and to make friends.

~

One momentous evening I overheard my older brothers discussing an alarming piece of news. Radio stations reported that some religious leaders declared Jesus would be returning that night for the faithful. My father dismissed the news; only God knew the hour of Christ's return he said, quoting the related scripture. I returned to my bed.

The evening train had long since rumbled by... yet I lay awake. Echoes of that long ago night of fireworks flashed across my mind. Except this night held a different sort of drama.

I pondered each page of the Wordless Book that my Sunday School teacher had given each of her students. I mentally rehearsed her explanation. Gold is for the promise of heaven and eternal life with God. Black is for my sinful disobedient nature inherited from Adam. Red is for the blood of Jesus shed on the cross to forgive my sin. White is for my heart made clean when I ask Him to forgive me and come in so He can wash me white as snow.

I also visualized the picture on my Sunday School paper of Jesus knocking on a heavy door with only one handle — on the inside. My mother had said that Jesus does not come in unless we decide to turn the handle and invite Him in.

I could no longer ignore this. Maybe Jesus would return that night and maybe not, but I still was not ready for Him. Knock, knock, went my heart. Tap, tap, came the patient gentle entreaty of the Lord upon my conscience. The time had come; I must decide.

Before the ten o'clock stroke of our clock, I pulled my covers off and knelt beside the bed on the cool hardwood floor. With head resting against folded hands I began: "Lord, I don't really understand how Your blood can make my heart clean but I know that if You do come back tonight I want to be ready to go with You. So I am asking You to forgive my sins, come live in my heart and make me Your child. Amen."

Rolling back under my sheets I waited for Him.

~

Sunshine streaming through the windowpane woke me up. I looked around. Why, nothing new had happened. Oh how deflating. Jesus had not returned. It appeared that my father and God's Word were right after all; no one could know the exact hour.

But as I dressed, ate breakfast and followed the dirt path to school, I began to realize that feelings had little to do with it. Something had happened all the same. Jesus had come. Not in the physical way I expected but He had come nonetheless.

In fact, I had turned the door handle to my heart and I would never need to wonder again about whether I was ready to meet Him. Now I could be certain that I belonged to Jesus; I had asked Him to come and live within me and I accepted His word that He did. At the time I did not realize that this sure conviction came from His indwelling Holy Spirit.

I could not prove it, but I had a new mindset. Regardless of my painfully shy and anxious nature, Jesus would help me to shine for Him. That was it: He wanted me to shine. That was my purpose and

I did not question it. "Jesus wants me for a sunbeam to shine for Him each day" — that was the chorus we sang at Sunday School. Simple. Straightforward.

~

My new bond with the Lord translated into a subtle but life-giving difference. Although I remained essentially self-conscious and challenged with schoolwork, I began to see my playmates as people whom Jesus wanted to include in His family as well. In my shy way I told them about how I had asked Jesus into my life.

At age ten I decided to be baptized before our church congregation as a sign of my union with Christ, along with my mother and cousin Linda. During recess I even gave a lively demonstration to my friends of how we had been dunked in the baptismal tank without being drowned. They laughed with me but I hoped they knew I loved Jesus and wanted to share His love for them, too.

~

chapter 2
Giddy schoolgirls, lonely aches, vulnerable sincerity

After one of my father's frequent business trips to the Toronto area, he made an announcement to our family. "How would you like to move to beautiful Oakville, Ontario?" His managerial skills were required at the company's Toronto office.

The year was 1958. I was eleven and eager for an adventure as were the rest of my siblings. Dad fed our imaginations with descriptions of the sprawling five-bedroom ranch home he and Mom bought — our first new home — in this prosperous bedroom community beside Lake Ontario. We were not disappointed. The towering pines in our front yard inspired Mom to name our home, *Whispering Pines*. Dad's eyes gleamed as he introduced us to the little Baptist church he had found for his large family. My father's instinct served us well; this congregation became our spiritual home for decades.

During a curious Christmas gift exchange I wondered if my Sunday School teacher had a good instinct as well. Mrs. Crawford had handed each eleven-year-old girl an envelope, explaining that she had given much thought and prayer to which type of gift each of us needed most. Inside we found a sentence or two intended just for us. It revealed to each girl what our teacher saw as our greatest asset. She asked us to keep the messages to ourselves and to consider how God meant us to use them.

I unfolded the paper, read the statement, and inwardly sighed. Was that all I was good for? Only that? *Elizabeth, your unique gift is your smile. God has given this to you for His glory.*

Only a smile. And yet, time has proven the godly wisdom and love this dear teacher had passed on to me in a simple revelation.

~

By age twelve, my interest focused on boys with the help of my Windsor cousin, Linda, whose family had moved to Oakville the same year we did. Giddy schoolgirls that we were, Linda and I — along with my grade seven companions, Donna and Sandy — tried to guess the kind of boy we would marry. We speculated about his name, his appearance, and romance in general, using one of those paper stars we folded and filled out with possible options for hair colour, eyes, height, occupation, number of children we would have and so on.

Our pastor was the last person I ever thought could supply us with a more reliable plan for our future than speculation and chance. When he visited our Pioneer Girls Club and suggested that God has a great interest in helping us find our future mates, my ears perked up. What did he mean?

Pastor Crawford said that if we let Him, God would help us to choose the marriage partner best suited for each of us. He assured us, "It is not too soon to start praying for that person now."

Although I was still interested in paper dolls, skipping ropes, and Hardy Boys mystery books, I took his suggestion to heart. In earnest I began to pray for that special someone wherever he was, asking God to show me His choice for me when the time came.

~

During this search for my own ideal man I developed many crushes, some based on charm and brawn, others on more substantial traits. I eventually met and dated a very nice boy through our church group who had both good looks and good character. Yet when we became engaged, this decision did not sit well in my spirit. Something was missing. For one thing I was too young at age eighteen for such a commitment. My family doctor, pastor and father all supplied the other answer I did not want to hear: this young man and I shared a similar melancholy temperament that would prevent a healthy balance.

After another year of ignoring their sound counsel and my own unease, I renewed my resolve to let God do my choosing. Recalling what my pastor had wisely recommended — to go home and ask God to show me His answer — I got down on my knees and promised God I would follow through on what He showed me. The answer couldn't be clearer; He had already given His direction through my adult mentors and my own doubts. I needed to break off the relationship so I could be available for God's best for me.

~

This most heartbreaking choice of my young life set the stage for me to trust God in much harder circumstances further down the road.

For a year I pined with loneliness. Would there ever be someone right for me and how would I recognize him? As I read scripture and prayed on a daily basis (habits I developed through the influence of my Sunday School teachers, Pioneer Girls Club, and my own Bible-reading parents) God gave me an insight that surprised and eased my lonely ache. In His mysterious way He assured my spirit that He had already set aside someone for me. I told God I did not know how I could care about someone else — it seemed like mutiny — but I decided to resume dating. I built new friendships through volunteer work at St. Christopher House in Toronto, part-time employment as a hospital ward aide, pumping gasoline at my dad's service station, plus Career and College events at our church.

How quickly I forgot God's promise that He would show me his choice. In the decade of the sixties young people were marrying in their early twenties. So as I approached my twenty-first birthday I worried that I might be too hard to please because none of the young men I met held my interest for long. My mother suggested I focus on my career and social life instead of fussing about whether I would find someone on time. She urged me to give myself another decade to mature, and expressed confidence that the right man would come along when I least expected it. Mom was right — but both of us were caught off guard by my next romantic encounter.

~

One evening while I was helping my mom to air out the cigar smoke left behind by brother Ken's best friend, Ron, my mother made a comment that left me aghast. "It would be good for you," she said, waving smoke out the window, "to marry a boy like him some day."

I stared at her. "Mom, you have got to be kidding! I would never consider someone like him – he is loud and arrogant!"

She ignored me. "That boy is exactly the kind of person you need." She pointed out that his confidence would counterbalance my timid tendencies.

Without another moment of consideration I brushed away Mom's suggestion as readily as the cigar smoke.

However, it would not be so easy to ignore the young man in question. Ron and I kept on bumping into one another under some hilarious circumstances, confirming my theory that God's ways do not exclude a sense of humour.

~

Aside from a civil nod I had never taken note of any friend my younger brother brought home because I assumed Ken's buddies would be too juvenile for me. How stuck up! However after a well-deserved rebuke from Ken about my snobbish ways and a surprise compliment from his buddy I began to pay more attention to this fellow. When Ron passed me in our front hallway, I caught him taking a second look at me in my new knit dress and heard him whistle something like "wow!" I was secretly tickled. Even if he did not appear on my radar of guys to date, an appreciative gesture felt good.

I made it my business to keep this fellow at arms length, but sometimes he was not so easy to dismiss.

When he and Ken crashed my recreation room birthday party with my closest friends and a new boyfriend, Ron offered me a birthday kiss to honour this 21st landmark. Eyes popping wide with dismay, I covered my mouth. No one was going to steal kisses that belonged to my future mate. Oh how my outburst seemed to amuse him! He smirked as he and Ken helped themselves to cake and let themselves out. Later when the other young man courting me asked me if he rated a kiss, I confessed that while I liked him I wasn't ready to make the kind of commitment that a kiss would imply.

No, I was not going to make it easy for any fellow who was interested in me. I was sincere about my commitment to that one chosen person but as far as I could tell he had not appeared yet so I wanted to keep my friendships casual. However I surprised myself and everyone else with my occasional cheek.

~

One Saturday evening I pulled into one of my dad's family-run service stations with a carload of girlfriends. We were heading for the Toronto Mutual Street Roller Rink. While Ken filled up the tank, his handsome sidekick stood at a distance observing us with his usual self-assured stance.

Recalling what I had recently heard about this Ron being a 'ladies' man', I announced to my friends, "Look at him, he thinks he's so cool. Watch this, girls!"

Driving up to where he stood, I rolled down my window and lifting my eyebrow, I said, "Hi…lover boy!"

My friends collapsed in shocked laughter, while I sped out of the lot before he could respond. My brothers' previous lessons in how to "burn rubber" came in handy for a quick getaway.

Incredulous, Ron turned to Ken and asked, "Who was that nervy chick?"

Ken chuckled, "Oh, that was only my sister". Well, that certainly amused Ron further because he hadn't recognized me. When Ken realized that his buddy's interest was piqued he said, "No way man. You do not want to go there — she's religious!"

Apparently up for a challenge, Ron asked me out. I consented on two conditions: that we double date with Ken and his girlfriend, and only three times. I made it difficult for this guy to even want that first date. I don't even remember why I wanted Ken along; maybe because I was not sure I was up to the challenges Ron might pose.

Sure enough, while riding in the back seat on our first chaperoned date, Ron tried to put his arm around me. My shoulders buckled like cracking ice. Ron quickly withdrew his arm before he got frostbite. Poor guy, I certainly did not intend to hurt his feelings. Nevertheless, we four had great times on our three outings — horseback riding, roller skating, and driving the scenic route to nearby Niagara Falls.

After our Niagara trip Ron joined me in my parents' kitchen for a late night cup of coffee and dessert. As I washed up the dishes, Ron hovered nearby quietly watching me. Oh, no, he is not going to ask me out again! He knows my rule about fourth dates.

But tonight his posture and his tone seemed different. I sensed a degree of vulnerable sincerity I had not picked up on during our dates. For me it had been an enjoyable experience, but a lark, that was all. I could not believe it when Ron asked me if I was willing to break my rule and go out again.

Thoroughly disarmed, I broke down and said yes.

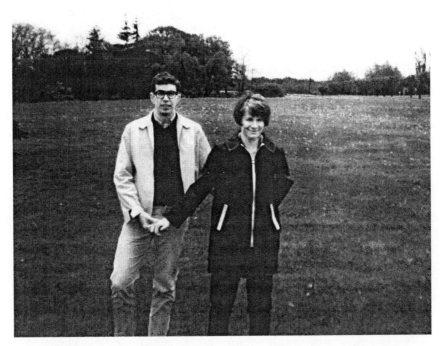

Our third date: falling in love against my will, Niagara Falls, 1968

He intrigued me; there seemed to be more depth to him than his surface cockiness. Maybe Ken was right when he had urged me to give his friend a fair chance after I had questioned his choice for best buddy. Just the fact that Ron wanted to bother knowing me better certainly indicated seriousness on his part since he had no shortage of female admirers. I was even willing to drop Ken as a prerequisite for our times together.

Through our conversations, long walks, movies and picnics, I found a great deal to admire. I grew to respect Ron's solid acceptance of himself, not allowing others to squeeze him into their moulds — including mine. I appreciated the way he listened to my ideas and acknowledged them while letting me know when he didn't agree.

23

I liked the gentlemanly way he treated me and other women of all ages, opening doors and bringing flowers to express appreciation or encouragement. I was warmed by his high regard for his mother. He thought the world of her for her tough-love loyalty to his alcoholic, gentle father. And I was impressed by Ron's compassionate spirit toward adolescent kids who were confused and lonely, offering them a shoulder and practical insights to get on with life.

Here was a man of character — someone I could look up to.

When his job as a hardware merchandiser took him out of town for a month Ron offered his birthstone ring as a symbol of our friendship. It seemed natural to accept the honour.

What did not make sense was the way my heart ached for his company during his absence and sprang to life whenever another post card arrived. He was, after all, a respected friend, not a sweetheart.

Then, while reading his third week of letters, I heard the rumble of a bass voice in the driveway. It sounded like Ron but his job didn't end for another week. I ran to the front door. And then I flew over the steps and along the driveway until I reached his car. Ken's best friend and now mine had returned early because he realized what I didn't know until then — our affectionate bond had turned into love.

~

This wasn't the way it was supposed to turn out! I thought I had guarded my heart against romantic entanglements. Hadn't I continued dating other fellows between my arms-length outings with Ron? So what had happened here? All I had done was honour Ken's request and it had backfired. Or had it?

Without a doubt Ron and I shared great chemistry and mutual respect. My mom was right – Ron's bold confidence balanced my insecure tendencies, while my gentleness offset his aggression. We both enjoyed the simple pleasures of walks and meaningful conversations with one another. But I needed a critical question answered.

Was this young man God's choice for me?

How could it be possible when Ron lacked one essential ingredient? He did not share my commitment to God. Although he had discontinued his drinking parties with Ken and attended church with me, this was not the same as following Christ. A marriage of two separate entities without dependence on the unifying Spirit of the Lord could be our undoing. We needed spiritual harmony. Unless that happened I could not envision a future for us together.

But, oh how I yearned to share it with this fine man!

~

In the quiet of my bedroom I promised God I would wait for Him to turn Ron's heart toward Him. Again that still small voice of God's Holy Spirit whispered peace. My panic settled. I received calm assurance that this would only be a matter of time. Had I misunderstood?

After dropping me off one evening, Ron sat in my parents' driveway absorbed in his own questions about our future. He knew that the way things stood I could not in good conscience marry him. What was he willing to do to win me over? God was not someone he had given much thought to. Sure, he believed someone had set the world in motion. He was even willing to call that creator "God" but not anything beyond that… he had often told me my faith was mere wishful thinking.

What happened next completely blindsided both him and me. Not until fifteen years later was I made privy to this moment, which I still remember with awe.

In the darkened hush of Ron's car a voice spoke to his heart, the way our conscience may alert us in an inaudible way, but Ron knew this was not coming from himself. This was the voice of God giving His beloved creation divine and practical insight. Graciously, the Spirit of the Lord spoke words of unmistakable confirmation: "This is the woman you are going to marry. You can trust her." Ron kept this revelation to himself.

Meanwhile, having not a clue of what had transpired, I held onto the Lord Jesus, my true hope and rest. When my trusted longtime friend Sharon rightly cautioned me about falling in love with a man who does not follow God, I replied that because I love Ron I want him to become a follower of Christ. Perhaps her prayers joined mine in storming heaven with urgency.

~

In my father's household, Sunday morning service was mandatory regardless of late nights and hangovers. For some time Ken had been dragging Ron along with him, both of them mostly dozing in the back pew. Then Ron began to attend church with me but I sometimes wondered what difference moving up a few pews might make. The message would still be the same. But one more message might mean everything when God is pursuing us, and breaking down our walls.

Pastor Crawford always delivered a hard-core message based on God's words to us in Scripture. At the closing hymn of each service his persuasive voice would call upon those who wanted prayer to raise their hands and/or come forward to the front altar as a resolve to follow Christ. Week after week since childhood I had thrilled to this holy opportunity when hungry hearts might acknowledge their need for the Shepherd of their souls and lives. God had planted in me this longing for others to let Christ set them free from their guilt and self-reliance. "Softly and tenderly Jesus is calling," we would sing and pray.

Imagine if you can what it meant that pivotal Sunday when the closing hymn began, "Just as I am without one plea, But that Thy blood was shed for me..." Stanza followed stanza.

Tension built with each line. "Just as I am though tossed about, with many a conflict, many a doubt... Just as I am, Thou wilt receive, wilt welcome, pardon, cleanse, relieve."

Oh Lord, I pleaded, *one of these days You will surely bring Ron to You.*

Sneaking a peak at the handsome young man seated near me, impeccably dressed in his trademark Harris tweed jacket and pressed slacks, I could note no change in his impervious demeanor. Many a conflict and doubt collided with my faith in God's faithfulness. The final chorus was winding down. For a moment I turned to my right as I noticed a person walk down the centre aisle. At the same time a movement ever so slight at my left arm caused me to look that way.

Ron stood up. Was he leaving?

No, the very opposite. He was heading purposefully down the left aisle. "O Lamb of God, I come! I come!" A long aisle but my beloved was striding to the front altar. We sang the final stanza again while our pastor laid his hand upon each person and prayed with him or her.

Dazed... incredulous... oh, can it be? I was trying to take in what was happening. I was watching this greatest of all miracles unfold. The heart of a man I was learning to love deeply, opening up to God. The hoped-for answer to a prayer was coming into view. Was this truly the beginning of Ron's walk with God, and our future as a couple?

Hadn't God promised me it would be only a matter of time? This was that time.

~

chapter 3
career quandary, May daze, baby bumps

As Ron grew in his faith so I did in mine and our love became sweeter. The details blur into a happy memory of courtship. Ron enjoyed showering me with flowers and small gifts and hugs and kisses, along with much laughter as I transformed into a willing recipient.

After seeking my parents' blessing, Ron asked for my hand in marriage on a July evening and slipped a silver engagement ring on my finger. We agreed to wait a year to marry giving us time to really get to know one another, and to allow me to complete my first year at Ryerson with the goal of becoming a social worker.

~

Although it did not seem like it at first, God was present in my career choice as well as in my life partner. After only five months into my course my field supervisor called me to her office. True, I found myself falling behind in my class assignments, yet I did not expect the advice she had for me. She recommended that I leave the course.

She did not believe my intense nature would be the best fit for this job, pointing out that I got too involved in the clients' dilemmas. She could not picture me leaving my work behind at the office at the end of the day. Neither could I.

Now what was I going to do? Through my late teens I had already explored the nursing option by working as a hospital ward aide full and part time for a few seasons. I knew that nursing was not what

I wanted, because I preferred more social interaction with patients than what that career allowed.

My supervisor said there was a 'however' in her news. I waited. She said she saw a place where she believed I would excel. She saw the skills of a teacher in me.

A teacher! Here it was again. This exact observation had been made years before by both my mom and my Pioneer Girls leader and mentor, Marge White.

Since my arrival at age eleven in her church, Marge had sensed God's calling to take me under her wing. Diligently she had developed my teaching abilities by enlisting and coaching me as her assistant in Junior Church classes. But I hadn't recognized any particular aptitude for teaching in myself. Aside from childhood efforts at subjecting my younger siblings to "lessons" in math and phonics on my birthday chalkboard, the idea of becoming a teacher had merely amused me.

However, since I was hearing the same thing from a neutral professional, perhaps it was time to take heed.

That day in late January when my dad picked me up from the GO train station and drove me home, I told him I was quitting school. Instead of expressing disappointment, he listened. How I appreciate the way Dad offered support for my decision even though he probably felt a sinking in his heart, wondering if I would ever follow through on my education.

~

Dad surmised my mind was preoccupied with my upcoming May wedding. He agreed that it seemed right to attend to that first. In time a career would unfold. With the help of my maid-of-honour sister, Susan, I shopped for my gown while my parents upgraded their bungalow for the big event.

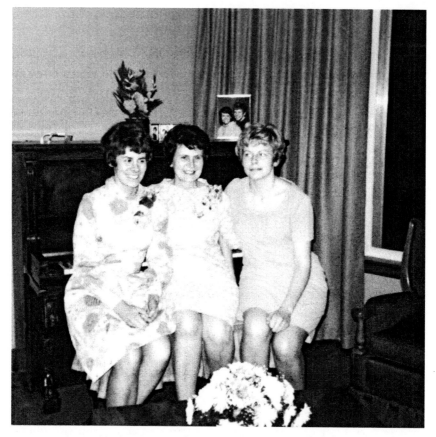

Mom, Susan and I enjoying my trousseau tea

Lovingly Mom and Susan helped plan my trousseau tea — a cultural tradition of the sixties — that preceded the wedding by a week. I wish I had been as relaxed for our wedding as I had been for this pre-party, displaying my honeymoon wardrobe and shower gifts.

When May 10, 1969 arrived I looked paler than my organza gown. Shaken with the prospect that the church would be packed with guests watching for the bride's entry, I decided a grand entrance had lost its appeal. I wanted to run down the aisle, say my vows, grab Ron and speed away. He agreed.

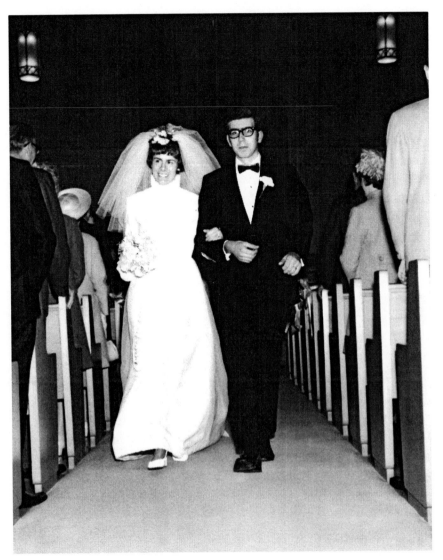

Yay, we're married! Oakville, 1969

My father ended our agony by keeping the dinner reception brief. After ninety minutes or so Dad rose and announced to the guests that the newly weds were eager to get off by themselves. His mischievous grin and twinkling eyes raised a ripple of laughter. Our guests clapped as we hurried away to begin our honeymoon. Ron's parents, my parents, siblings, and wedding party saw us off at the side door of the church. My lovely sister Susan beamed for our happiness.

But where was Ken? We half expected him to pop up in the back seat of our car wearing a silly grin and eager to chaperone us as he had done in the beginning. As we drove off Ron turned on the air vents; confetti flew like feathers around us. "Ken!" we both laughed — the culprit!

If a person were to predict the success of a marriage by the reticence our wedding day evoked in us, we would have been sunk because neither Ron nor I felt comfortable with the focus on us. Like our wedding we kept our Ottawa honeymoon short, especially when we woke up to thick snow covering the tulips outside our motel window. We packed up and headed back to Burlington. What we wanted most was to slip, undetected, into our town and begin life in our own cozy three-story walkup on Lakeshore Boulevard.

"Mrs. Morgan, may I?" my groom asked.

My romantic Ron swept me over the threshold of our new life together.

Oh how I enjoyed the sound of my new name: "Mrs. Morgan, Mrs. Ron Morgan". Married life fit me like a doeskin glove. Ron attentively wanted to give me priority, still courting me with long walks, flowers and sweet words. We were warned that sooner or later the bloom would fade. So we decided never to take each other for granted.

~

My enrollment in Teacher's College that autumn tested our resolve. I worked long into the night preparing assignments and lessons while my love went to bed alone, learning how to give me room to work. It must have been a lonely first year for Ron. There were times when I doubted whether God was calling me to this career; I was not a quick study, never was. After one stressful week of practice teaching in an enrichment grade eight class I was blindsided by the training teacher's advice. His bottom line: *You are not a teacher. You should quit while you're ahead.*

There it was again; a professional telling me what I was not cut out for! I went home and dropped my bomb. Ron was not impressed that I was quitting.

He urged me to return for one more day to teach my Friday lesson, giving it all I had to give, even if I had to stay up all night. After a heated protest I agreed to do that, setting my despair aside. What had I to lose? To alleviate my grief Ron pointed out that from what I had already told him about this supervisor, he might not be the most qualified judge to direct my career.

Armed with dynamic lessons and a surge in confidence I walked back into the class ready to give my best performance. Halfway through the first lesson, a visitor arrived and sat down with my supervising teacher. He wasn't just any visitor. He was one of the professors from my Teacher's College who arrived to mark my progress. What might have rattled me at an earlier time now left me with a so-what attitude.

So what if the top dog appraises me? So what if I'm going down? I might as well go down with guns blazing. The visitor stayed until recess, jotting notes as he observed my techniques and material. After I dismissed the children, I joined the two men for my beheading.

Point by point my professor went through my lessons giving his assessments while I sat waiting for the boom. It eventually came but it was beyond anything I had anticipated.

"Mrs. Morgan," (oh I still liked hearing my newly acquired name even though I expected to have my career dreams dashed again) "I find that not only are you a good teacher... you are an outstanding teacher."

Wait a minute. I looked at the training teacher and thought, *but yesterday he said... and then at my professor, but you just said...*

What a different tune! The truth probably lay between the two poles. When I returned home that evening Ron asked how things had gone. He was over the top when he heard the second opinion.

"Hon, I knew that first opinion was not to be taken seriously. What do you want to do next?"

Together we discussed options. Ron said that whether or not teaching turned out to be my thing, it was still important to finish the course for my own morale. He cautioned me not to quit prematurely, leaving with a sense of defeat. The goal became to finish what I had started.

After a year of toughing it out, I claimed my prized teaching certificate with my proud husband, mom, sister, and mom-in-law cheering me on in the audience. My beloved Ron deserved to share that achievement with me; he had endured lonely nights of neglect while my attention was riveted on work. He took a back seat for a time, while my learning difficulties required full focus.

We grads were advised that since teaching positions were severely limited we ought to move on to another career if we did not immediately land a teaching job. I decided to pursue my permanent teaching certificate by substitute teaching to accumulate the two mandatory years. This meant I was observed and marked by the principal of every school I taught in, to verify my qualifications.

During these teaching days on my own I developed a repertoire of lessons for every grade and subject — kindergarten to grade eight — plus a bag of tricks to ensure that learning took place in an atmosphere of fun and accountability. Not wanting to be a mere babysitter in the home teacher's absence I grew into a professional substitute teacher, thanks to the tips and encouragement of Ron and my longtime mentor Marge, also a substitute teacher.

~

During these early years of our marriage Ron and I enjoyed weekend hikes on the Bruce Trail or leisurely bike rides and picnics along picturesque Lakeshore Road, following the shore of Lake Ontario from our apartment in Burlington to neighbouring Oakville.

Ron and I also kept busy as leaders in church-sponsored boys and girls clubs as well as our young married class. Ron developed his considerable aptitude for retail management and inventory control, working his way up in the hardware store industry while I continued as an on-call teacher to Halton County schools, combining our earnings for Ron's dream of owning his own hardware franchise some day.

Agreeing with what my mom had quietly advised me about not starting a family right away, we decided to give ourselves a few years to relish our time alone. After nearly three years we were ready to add to our twosome.

A few months later I felt quite rundown so I visited our family doctor who ordered some basic tests. When he called me to return for a second visit I hoped he had not found something amiss.

"Dr. McGee" assured me nothing was wrong… unless I did not want a baby yet. "A baby! You mean I'm already pregnant?"

"Liz, my girl," he clapped me on the back, "you and Ron have made your first child."

I couldn't wait to tell Ron! Oh, how I loved him. It still amazed me that I had fallen for him so gradually, unexpectedly, and profoundly.

~

I planned to make the announcement through a clever poem at Ken's twenty-fifth birthday party that same evening.

My mother had invited the extended family over for the surprise dinner celebrations. Ron was supposed to deliver Ken home at the designated time. I envisioned Ron reading my poem privately with me — and then we would declare the good news to everyone. Instead we listened to my parents' mantel clock chiming eight gongs, nine gongs, then ten. When the delinquent pair finally arrived, wearing sheepish grins on greasy faces, we were too annoyed to sympathize with their excuses about forgetting the time while fixing Ken's racing car.

As Ron and I drove to our own apartment I sat in silence hugging the passenger door.

"Hon, I'm really sorry for spoiling the party." He patted the space next to him. "Come on Liz, move over here closer to me."

After nearly three years of marriage my husband still knew how to butter me up. But this night I wasn't budging. My family's surprise had been spoiled — and so had mine, but of course he didn't know about that part.

Ron wondered how to appease me. After a while he withdrew as well. Misery hung between us.

Suddenly he remembered my errand earlier in the day. "So what did Dr. McGee say about your tiredness?"

I couldn't help myself; I smiled in the darkness of our old station wagon. With as much nonchalance as I could muster I answered, "Oh nothing much, you know, the usual thing."

"Well what was that, Hon? Explain." Ron's voice was edged with impatience.

With a sideways glance I watched his response as I delivered the news. "Oh, all he said was that… you're going to be a daddy."

"He said WHAT???"

Before I knew it, my sweetheart had squealed the car onto the shoulder of Lakeshore Road and pulled me into his arms.

"This is great Hon! You and I are going to have a baby! Oh I love you so much, Liz!"

Yes, I knew that. We were friends, lovers and partners for life. And we were wonderfully happy together; having a baby provided one more blessing to share.

~

Family and friends commented that they had never seen me looking so well. Ron and I both glowed with anticipation. Nausea could not suppress my high spirits. But toward the fourth month as my slender frame began to swell with promise, I developed a mysterious symptom.

The first time it happened I was coming home at dusk from my teaching job. We were climbing up the stairs to our apartment.

"Ron, I need help."

"What's the matter? Why are you stopping on the stairway?"

"I don't know what just happened but my knees are locked." My legs remained frozen in mid-step.

My husband had to carry me up our three-story walk-up. Over many days this incident repeated itself. I was okay on level ground but by evening I couldn't manage the climb. Joint pain awoke me most nights. My brother Bill and mother both had the genetic disease, rheumatoid arthritis. Could this be happening to me as well?

Alarmed, I finally revisited our family doctor who ordered standard blood tests. He concluded my problems stemmed from urinary tract infection and suggested an antibiotic.

I considered that since I rarely took aspirin let alone a stronger drug, I was reluctant to take something that might harm our baby.

Peering over thick glasses, Dr. McGee regarded me with amused candour. "Liz, Liz, you worry too much."

"I know but I don't want anything to happen," I said touching my abdomen. Was the medication necessary or would it be okay to forgo it?

Dr. McGee reflected, "Look, you only have a low-grade infection... we'll let the infection run its course." Clapping me on the back in his fatherly way, he sent me on my way.

Down the road Ron and I wished we had been informed of the risks this decision involved. We could have been spared much lifelong trauma but being a novice patient I did not know the right questions to ask, and missed out on critical information my physician could have given me.

By the fifth month the symptoms of stiff joints subsided as mysteriously as they had appeared. We assumed that an infection caused the problem and had run its course as the doctor predicted. We could rest easy.

~

We enjoyed our role as parents-in-waiting. Carefully we documented each month's progress, ensuring a healthy regimen for myself with plenty of fresh air, rest, and a balanced diet. I taped Canada's Food Rules to a kitchen cupboard door. Our frequent camping trips to the sand dunes of The Pinery became a refreshing health ritual.

My husband even helped me monitor the amount of stress I was exposed to, reasoning that my emotional well-being would affect the baby's health as well. This meant that I only accepted teaching jobs in the lower grades where children were easier to manage. I limited social contacts to positive people.

By the time the October winds of 1972 had whipped the last leaves from the trees around our apartment building, the baby furniture had been painted aqua, walls papered and linoleum installed in the spare room. A generous shower given by my family filled our baby dresser with newborn outfits. I even washed the delicate things in Ivory Snow to ensure that the manufacturer's chemicals would not touch our child's skin.

There was nothing left to do but pack my suitcase with the peach and pale blue baby sets, knit by Ron's Aunt Dee Dee. And wait for the enormous luggage around my middle to make its move.

When Ron and Ken returned from the Sunday evening service on November 12th I informed them that it was time. Feigning calmness they tripped over one another trying to grab the suitcase and start the car. Excitement collided inside of me, too while my body prepared to release the child. Although I didn't think so at the time, labour progressed smoothly. Down the hallway from my labour room I heard a woman who screamed non-stop.

"Someone please shut that woman up," I snapped, not expecting the pain to be this pervasive.

Having heard horrific labour stories from one of my mother's dramatic friends, but knowing my mom had gone through this seven times without voicing any complaints, I made an erroneous conclusion that this would be a breeze. The truth hovered somewhere inbetween. My fellow labourer was merely giving in to what I desperately wanted to do. My husband showed great forbearance as he closed the door so that I could focus on the Lamaze breathing method of controlling pain. My months of practice paid off. I never hyperventilated nor lost my place but I promised myself — and Ron — "Never again!" Never would I go through this again!

Six hours later my tune changed when I wept with ecstasy as Ron and I took turns cradling our beautiful son. Bring on the babies; I wanted more.

Transferred to the maternity ward to rest, I could not sleep. I pulled the heavy drapes back from the window, surprised to see the late autumn sky filling with flakes — the first snowfall of the season — and marvelled at the freshness of new things. Snuggling back under my covers, I drifted off…. How exquisite it felt to be a mother.

Suddenly the ward came alive as lights switched on and tiny bundles were delivered to their respective moms for feeding time.

Since no one brought my baby I rolled over for another well-earned sleep. No doubt, the nurses wanted me to recover strength before breastfeeding my baby for the first time.

Before long, lights once more pierced my eyelids and babies squalled. I sat up watching for a nurse to bring baby Mark to me. I wondered if I would be able to recognize him from all the others.

But my baby never came.

~

Instead a nurse stopped at my bedside with a pen and paper. "Mrs. Morgan, a little problem has developed with your baby. We need you to sign a release form for your son, Mark."

"Problem?" I was trying to remember the way my firstborn looked lying in the crook of my arm… chubby and adorable… my heart bursting with speechless joy. But what was it about his tummy that vaguely disturbed me… something strange in its appearance… was it my imagination or was it distended and green?

Yet none of the staff had commented about it so there was apparently nothing to worry about. Normal stuff for newborns, I presumed.

The nurse continued, "Your baby has a problem that will require surgery… "

She didn't get to finish. Dr. McGee breezed past her, dragged the green curtain around me and sat down.

Coke-bottle glasses falling low on his nose he looked me directly in the eyes. I could always count on Dr. McGee to get to the point. "Liz, your son has been born with what we call an 'umbilical hernia'. We have to transport him to Sick Children's Hospital in Toronto. This morning. I'm sorry. I'll call Ron." He left as abruptly as he arrived.

Whoosh. Just like that my euphoria had been whisked away.

The nurse returned to complete her task. She explained that the green bulge I had noticed on Mark's abdomen was actually his bowel covered by a film of skin. Since specialists didn't know at what stage in the pregnancy the hernia developed they could not predict whether there would be room in the stomach cavity to return the bowels. "Risky surgery," they said. They might need to create a bag outside his abdomen and do a series of surgeries over time to make room for the intestines.

I stared at the nurse, stared at the form, signed on the dotted line and watched her hurry off with the legal document.

I lay back against my pillow while my eyes followed the swirling flakes. The day that had begun with promise mocked me now.

"Flowers for the new mom," a ward aide announced as she brought me a bouquet of red roses. I read the sweet note attached to the bundle. What would my Ron say when the doctor called him about this turn of events? I pictured how he would reassure me that it would all work out, that our son would come through.

As soon as Ron received the call he came to my side. My strong, consistently practical husband fell into my arms weeping; together we wept for the child our love had produced.

Bringing a newborn into the world and then consenting to that helpless little one's surgery elicited emotions never experienced before. As the hours passed and other parents cuddled their babies, we waited for further news. At last a nurse approached us, her face not registering the nature of her report. We were ready for anything — the worst and the best. Just tell us.

"Sick Children's Hospital just called." Apparently the hernia occurred late in the pregnancy meaning that the bowel cavity had not closed in with the other organs. The surgeon was able to drop the intestines back in with no problem.

Hoping we understood correctly, Ron and I exchanged glances and looked back at her.

"Your son is going to be alright."

We silently breathed a prayer of thanksgiving to God for sparing our baby more complications.

We were told that Mark would need to stay at the hospital a few weeks until he recovered and then he could come home.

While I remained in the Oakville Hospital for the standard week, Ron drove daily into the prestigious Toronto Sick Children's to hold our son. He took pictures of Mark for me to see. The staff provided a rocking chair where he could rock and feed our baby the breast milk I was sending along.

When I was released from hospital it felt unreal to return home without carrying a baby in my arms. Yet when the news came that Mark had recovered so well that we could take him home earlier than expected, we both felt something close to panic.

~

Gulp. This was the real thing. We were now fully responsible for nurturing this little life we had hoped and prayed for. What did we know about caring for an infant, let alone the broader task of parenting? We would muddle through with the help of instinct, love and our experienced moms.

Our cozy twosome would be taxed by the demands of our sturdy new member who knew how to make our nerves stand on end with every fretful cry. Was he okay? Should we let him cry? Our doctor said not to give in; your son is fully recovered, let him learn who is boss. But Ron and I took turns tiptoeing into Mark's room after he stopped crying to make sure he was still breathing. We knew better! That little guy would start up again and we would be beating our chests. Finally we made a pact to help one another wait it out each night. Our insides churned, but after one month our Mark finally settled down and slept.

~

During the New Year's party we held in our apartment we showed off our six-week-old cutie and then rocked him to sleep. But babies being clever little creatures — no one as clever as one's own offspring, of course — ours decided to test the waters again. He began to cry for more attention. No one came. Then he stopped and listened. Hmmm, he must have thought... I better cry a little louder. Sure enough! Ron and I caught both of our mothers converging at the hallway leading to their grandson's bedroom door. We cut them off at the pass and corralled them back into the living room. They shrugged sheepishly knowing that we had already worked hard to acquire a measure of competence as first time parents.

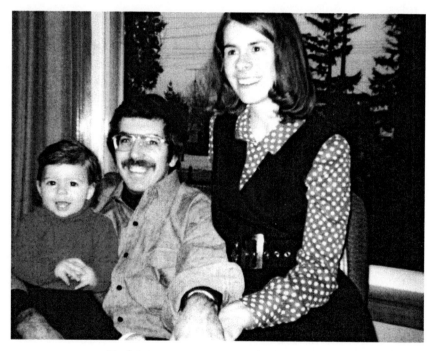

Mark joins our twosome, Burlington 1972

~

chapter 4
compassionate presence, patronizing tone, surprise conclusion

Mark's surgery proved successful, enabling him to develop into a healthy sociable toddler. So much so that he started cutting the apron strings as soon as he could crawl. A Canadian flag sown on the back of a jean jacket was often spotted by neighbours as our toddler jetted by, in search of playmates in our townhouse complex. Ron and I enjoyed parenting our youngster, strapping him to his dad's back for camping trips and picnic hikes along the Bruce Trail.

But I felt a growing uneasiness about my own health. Although my stiffness had vanished by the second trimester, weakness and nausea continued to plague me long after Mark's birth. I asked the doctor to retest my blood.

"The sediment rate is low and that means you have a low-grade infection." Nothing to worry about, he said.

"I thought that problem resolved itself a long time ago! Is this why I'm weak and weepy all the time?"

"You gave birth to a baby… give it time… you'll feel better."

No, he's wrong, I argued inside. *Enough time has passed.*

Why was I still dragging myself from one day to the next? By now I should feel better. While normally healthy women returned to their careers, I had little stamina. I couldn't even manage a morning of home chores, sleeping whenever our youngster had his catnaps.

The conflict within me continued. *He's the doctor; he knows the score. Be a good patient and don't disagree.* Yet I couldn't erase the unease.

The lethargic symptoms intensified. More tests revealed the alarmingly familiar presence of infection.

"What is causing this infection? Where is it located? Why does it keep showing up?" I demanded answers.

Dr. McGee assured me that although he could not locate its source there was nothing to worry about, as long as it remained low-grade. I wanted to believe him. After all, I was just a patient while he had trained for years to give me his professional opinion.

Since 'nothing was wrong' I pushed myself to resume an active lifestyle. While Mark's Grandma Morgan cared for him I resumed my on-call teaching job, often returning home physically and emotionally wrung out. Coming home to Ron and Mark — who were both my joys — did not remove the fatigue. When I asked to see specialists, Dr. McGee humoured me with referrals.

The experts agreed with him — my symptoms of fatigue stemmed from stress and nothing more. There was nothing for me to do but live with the professional consensus: to get beyond these symptoms and carry on with my multiple roles as wife, mother, on-call teacher and Pioneer Girls guide.

Always eager to help me roll with the stuff life throws at us, Ron would think of ways to do that. One time he brought me a *Holly Hobby* cloth calendar for our kitchen wall. The verse on it reminded me of a winning attitude to nurture. It said: *Now is the time to be happy.*

How very apt. What was the point of stalling in self-pity when life offered good things every day regardless of the troubles? I asked God to show me the beauty He sends in a day — the way my child beamed whenever his crayon drawing was displayed on the fridge door, or the way my husband would call me in the middle of his workday to tell me he loves me, or the way sunlight drew patterns on a wall.

~

When I seemed to rally, we decided it would be good to have children close in age – two or three years apart seemed reasonable. By the start of '74 a second pregnancy occurred and we began to antici-pate the joy of adding to our family unit.

On a late March morning a neighbour and I were planning an outing when I mentioned that I had passed some blood. She urged me to lie down. I was disturbed with the fuss but since she was a nurse I decided to heed her concern. Cramping followed soon after. Several hours later Ron checked me into the emergency ward.

A young specialist spoke softly to ease my tension. "It looks like your body is trying to abort the fetus. You are at twelve weeks, a stage when spontaneous abortions are common."

"What are you going to do?" I whispered, twisting one corner of my sheet but too stunned to weep.

"We're going to see if labour pains will stop in the next five hours or so. If not… well, rather than letting you suffer needlessly we will take the fetus by a simple procedure called a 'D&C'." As he left the room he squeezed my foot.

I wished I had not insisted that Ron return to work until I called for him. We did not expect this to be a big deal. The tiny room was white, sterile and cold. There was nothing to offer comfort — no tiny plaque or picture to focus on, no friend to hold my hand. I should call for Ron to come back but there was something stubbornly inde-pendent in my nature.

~

Although I was alone, I became aware of a great Compassionate Presence, as though Someone were stroking away my last reserve. My carefully controlled emotions melted away. First tears came in drops then in streams. As I wept freely a simple children's chorus ran through my mind… *Jesus loves me this I know.* Beyond a shadow of a doubt I knew in that aching moment that Jesus ached with me. His comfort was as solid as the table I lay on.

Labour pains strengthened by the hour. The decision was simple. As the gynaecology surgeon passed my stretcher in the Operating Room corridor he stopped for a moment and with his hand wiped my silent tears. When I awoke from surgery and knew for certain that the tiny inert baby in me was removed, grief squeezed my maternal soul. This was my initiation into the world of loss, and the wound went deep.

Ron caressed my fingers as I came out of surgery. We thanked God that during my recovery, the gentle hands of a former class-mate and head nurse of the ward washed me and wiped my tears. My dad came to my bedside and in his reserved way took my hand in his gnarly one. Although Dad could not verbalize his sorrow, I knew he hurt with me.

Likewise for my dear mom-in-law who wanted to comfort me by telling me this was 'nature's way'. I had already been told that several times and though I knew it was true it did not address my loss. When I told Mom this was not what I needed to hear right now she began to weep with me. It was what we both needed. This was her loss too — a potential grandchild. Upon my discharge another nurse, a lively sociable woman, wheeled my chair to the elevator. While we waited for a car, she seemed at first to be immune to my grief as she chattered non-stop to another staff member. Yet her heart was very much aware… she combed my hair with her fingers as they talked.

How sweetly strangers and loved ones had touched our word-less sorrow.

~

A few days after I left the hospital I took Mark for a walk to the park. It was a glorious sunny morning. Perching my precious brown-eyed boy on my lap I began to push the swing away from the ground climbing higher with every thrust. Mark shrieked with delight. For a while the rushing air brushed away my sadness and as we swung I composed a song to swing by:

Wouldn't you like to go high
Way, way, way up to the sky
Just hop on a swing
And spread out your wings
And see how high you can fly?

Mark sang along with me, happy to see his mommy smiling again. A second verse followed. Although the ache within felt immense, I couldn't let it rule me. There were other people in my life needing my care.

Ron gave me comfort and support with flowers, and prayers, often taking Mark to the park so I could rest. In turn I wanted to give my husband what he needed too. I determined to surmount this new loss by focussing on all I still had to be grateful for.

~

Two years after that miscarriage I delivered a second robust son, Paul — another delight for my maternal soul and our family. A low maintenance baby, he preferred sleeping to waking every few hours for feedings. By the third month Paul was diagnosed with a visual impairment that required glasses as soon as he was able to keep them on. By age two Paul was outfitted with bifocals to aid his sight. Although he squinted in sunlight our determined son managed to find his way around the neighbourhood and later in the classroom, never willing to draw attention to his poor vision.

What fun to watch the complementary temperaments in our sons – one eager to dash off and the other to snuggle.

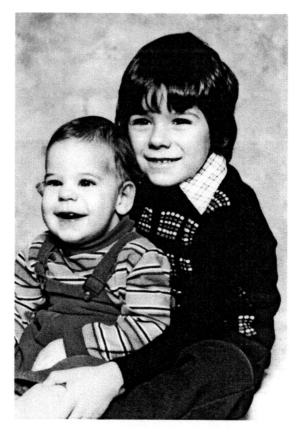

Paul, a baby brother for Mark, Burlington, 1976

We loved to spend time with them on picnics, bike hikes and soccer games but we also recognized the need to nurture our relationship as a couple.

In order to keep our romantic spark alive, Ron planned regular dates and special hideaway weekends for the two of us at *Prudhomme's*, a recreation centre and hotel an hour or so from home. Time would prove this to be a priceless investment for our marriage and family life.

A year after Paul's arrival I experienced fatigue with a double vengeance. By playing mind games I tried to convince myself that two active youngsters justified my feelings of burnout.

~

But a disquieting voice within me whispered ominous forecasts: *Something's wrong, something's still wrong. Listen to your body; listen to your instinct.*

Throughout those trying years my husband endured my mood swings with infinite patience, but I wondered when he would throw up his hands in despair. Although Ron struggled to understand the cause of symptoms he surely suspected psychosomatic reasons. What else would he believe after eight years of undiagnosed symptoms?

Finally he addressed the matter. "Hon, I have to tell you that you're not yourself. Your personality has changed."

I trembled. Would my practical spouse tell me to smarten up and take control of my emotions or else…?

"At first I thought you were experiencing stress," Ron admitted, "but you're getting worse. There must be a logical reason the doctors have overlooked." Raising a clenched fist, Ron resolved, "Hon, we will go after those guys until they find out what's wrong."

We discussed my options. I could return to my family doctor and push him for real answers or find another physician.

"Dear Dr. McGee," I wrote, "I appreciate the kindness you have shown me over the years — yet I feel that you have failed to take me seriously. I need someone who will listen with a fresh perspective." It grieved me to leave my family doctor but I needed to pursue a different course for the sake of my family.

And for my own sake, too. Verdicts of stress and nothing more had eroded my morale and confidence.

~

On a warm day two months later I lay shivering under a paper sheet waiting for the new family doctor to give his professional opinion. During previous weeks he had conducted a series of tests and personal interviews about my history.

"Dr. Clark" knocked and entered the room holding a sheaf of papers. Kind eyes viewed me under bushy eyebrows. "Liz, I don't think there is anything physically wrong with you."

My spirits thudded to the floor.

"What about my symptoms?"

"There's no doubt that you are feeling ill…."

There it was: that patronizing tone, the way he said 'feeling'. I already knew that old song and dance.

"But I believe those symptoms would go away if… well, if you had more faith. Liz you worry too much."

If I had more faith? Now there was a new theme. What did he know about my faith? I had heard he was a devout believer in God, but he had no business judging my level of faith. If someone would find out what was wrong, then I would stop worrying!

I wanted to shout all those things at him and walk out. But that would have made an undignified exit since my clothes lay at the foot of the examining table. Instead I kept my mouth shut and listened to the rest of his advice.

Combing fingers through his greying moustache, he continued, "I recommend you go for counselling which I will be glad to provide in the evenings or…."

I finished the sentence for him, "Or I can see a psychiatrist?"

He nodded with an apologetic expression.

~

Ron was more outraged than I that the new doctor would suggest I was lacking in faith.

For the next month I wrestled with myself and with God, pouring out my agony into my journal of prayer. True, I was a worrier, but without my faith in the Lord I would be lost. I chided myself for pretending at a faith in God which perhaps I had never possessed at all. All those wasted years feeling sick when it was my own spiritual and mental health at risk… all those wasted years of thinking doctors were wrong and I was right.

However I decided not to subject myself to Dr. Clark's well-intentioned counsel let alone a psychiatrist. I had heard plenty of horror stories from friends whose minds and lives ended up in a deeper mess after exposure to inept psychiatrists. Somehow I would carry on with my busy life, ignore my fatigue and growing nausea, and find the means to develop more substantial faith.

As often as possible I searched for spiritual rest, sitting on the sunny front steps of our townhouse during quiet morning times with my Bible and prayer journal in hand. Would this be enough?

~

It was an autumn day in November of '81. A big day for our Mark — his ninth birthday! We made plans to celebrate with a party at Fort York on the following day, Saturday. Meanwhile I had sandwiches and a cake to prepare, as well as taking time for a rest after lunch.

Seven am. The phone jarred my focus. The voice asked, could I get to a school ten miles across town by 8:30 to teach a grade five class? Oh, why today! I should have declined so I would be fresh for the special event, but I ignored my mounting weariness and said yes.

"Come on guys, step on it!" I called. "We have only half an hour to get you two off to school and the sitter."

Mark shrugged his shoulders and continued to doddle. I became incensed. Before I knew it I had sent his slender frame reeling across the kitchen floor.

I couldn't believe what was happening. I had just thrown my child against the baseboard. Who was this violent woman?

I stood rooted to the spot, staring at the bright magnet birds on our fridge door, and clawed my hands through my hair. Then I heard a scream... again and again more screams. Chilling high-pitched screams.

Mark's gentle brown eyes stared in horror. "Mom, Mom, don't do that!" he begged.

His brother retreated to the hallway.

I must stop this. It's Mark's birthday. I must stop.

As though I were watching a film I saw my body crumple onto the floor beside Mark. I heard pitiful sobs coming from myself — and from my birthday boy. Where was God in all of this? How could I have done this to one of my boys!

Abruptly I stopped. Got up. And quietly instructed Mark to walk Paul to the sitter's place and continue on to school.

Then I called my gynaecologist to say that I was admitting myself to the psych ward at the hospital. She assured me I had had a bad moment but not to be so hard on myself. She advised me to suspend all activities for the day and consider my next plan of action for better health.

The following day we carried on with the promised fort party.

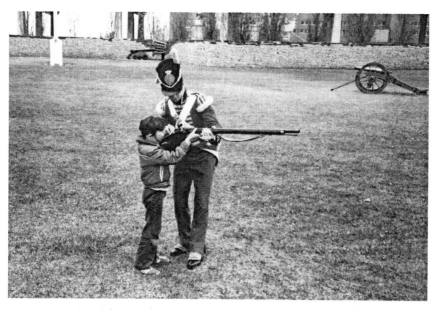

Mark has birthday party at Fort York, Toronto, 1981

Mark and his friends enjoyed their experience as they helped with the loading and firing of cannons, and later ate peanut butter sandwiches, cake and ice cream in an actual fort barrack.

~

After discussing my violent behaviour and increasing fatigue, Ron and I chose two critical steps to move us beyond the current limbo. We made the decision we had earlier balked at; I would submit myself to psychiatric care. This time we did not need convincing.

The choice of which doctor also became a matter of prayer and waiting on God to make the way clear. A name was presented to us through a close friend who worked for a psychiatrist she respected. We proceeded with the assumption that God would honour our measure of trust — the size of a mustard seed but enough in His hands.

We also addressed my outburst by gathering our boys around the kitchen table and explaining that it wasn't their fault what had happened. I asked their forgiveness and told them I was not well and needed to rest a lot. Ron promised our sons the right doctor would help their mom get better.

~

In the midst of these uncertain times, our boys provided us with many uplifting moments to amuse or warm our spirits.

On a lazy Sunday afternoon, I asked Paul to get his dad up from his nap. Paul returned. "I told Daddy that he should get up and Daddy said, 'okay.'"

"So, is he getting up?" I pressed.

"Yes," my five-year-old said. "But first he's going to have a *sleep*, then he's going to have a *nap*, and then he's going to have *a rest*."

I laughed and laughed at Paul's accurate observation of his father's napping habits. I heard Paul telling nine-year-old Mark in the next room, "Mommy's being silly."

I laughed even harder.

Later that afternoon, Ron told me that Mark and Paul had snuggled into bed with their father, one on either side of him.

Mark must have been contemplating something he heard in Sunday School because he remarked to his waking dad, "You're my daddy but you're my brother too, because we're both Christians."

Those are moments that choked us up.

~

I scanned the foyer board listing the offices.

DR HAYNES PSYCHIATRIST ROOM 304.

Taking deep breaths I rode the elevator up. A nurse promptly ushered me into the doctor's presence. My palms gripped the arms of the leather chair. A small man in his mid-40's smiled kindly at me; indulgently, I thought, like all the rest of his kind.

I examined him as carefully as he examined me. Could I trust him? My friend trusted "Dr. Haynes" as her employer but she had never been his patient. Undoubtedly he wondered into what degree of insanity I had slipped. That was his job, wasn't it, to assess my mental condition?

"Tell me, Mrs. Morgan, why are you here?"

"I don't want to be here!" I retorted. "This office is the last place I want to be." I glared at the foot of his desk and then at him. His face — an ordinary face — registered no response to my hostility.

He waited.

"Well, I guess I'm here because my GP sent me here."

"Go on."

"For ten years I have been ignored by GPs and specialists. No one believes me that I am ill. A year ago I switched to a new family doctor and he doesn't believe me either. He insists there is no physical cause for my symptoms. He just thinks I am overwrought and need psychiatric help."

"And... what do *you* think?"

"I've always known that something is seriously wrong. But now I don't know what to believe any more. I'm beginning to suspect that I *am* sick in the head... like they suggest." Images of magnet birds and insane behaviour hovered near.

Dr. Haynes began to rummage in his drawer until his hands found what he was searching for. Across his desk he arranged his smoking accessories: pipe, several bags of tobacco, box of matches and a stoke. With unhurried movements he filled his pipe, lit it, puffed a few times to get it started and leaned back to savour his smoke.

As I watched him follow this ritual with obvious satisfaction, I felt the knots in my neck ease up.

Finally he glanced up as though he had just remembered I was still there.

"Mrs. Morgan, why don't you begin by telling me what has been happening to you over the last ten years: your symptoms, your family and your marriage… whatever comes to mind." Turning his chair away from me he continued his long slow draws on his pipe while staring out the open window.

What did this small man with bad teeth care about one more recital from one more patient? Well, I didn't care much either. I'd say my piece and then get out of there. So, where should I begin? One thing for sure — this man was not going to hear about my family and my life. I was not here for that psychobabble. I came to address my symptoms and that's all he was going to hear about.

Little did I realize that it would not end that neatly.

Not only did he want to hear my life story, Dr. Haynes asked me to return for weekly appointments. He seemed genuinely committed to finding the root of my problem as he probed further into my childhood, marital and medical background, including standard blood and urine tests as a part of his investigation.

When he broached the topic of my faith, I thought, *oh brother, here we go!* I was aware that some mental illness could present itself as fanatically religious, the patient even believing himself to be a deity like God. I told him about my belief in Jesus my friend and Lord, urging him not to undermine the one thing that keeps me going. The doctor nodded, then he asked me if I could *see* Jesus. I said that I often place Jesus in an empty chair near me when I find myself in a situation where I feel intimidated or uncomfortable — "like right now in this office," I added.

Gently, the doctor nodded toward the two other empty chairs in his office. "Show me which chair He's sitting in… where do you see Him?"

I laughed. "Oh, I can't see where He is. I just mentally place Him in this chair nearest to me," I said as I touched the padded chair on my right, "to give me comfort."

I explained that Jesus has promised His followers that "He will never leave us nor forsake us" so I trust that God's spirit is nearby. It seems that the doctor was satisfied with my answer because the matter never came up again.

I breathed a prayer of thanks to God that He had not granted me the answer I had requested a few months earlier. When questioning God's seeming absence from solutions for my mysterious illness I had entreated Him: would He physically appear to me for a moment to assure me that He really does exist as He has done at different times in the history of mankind? By not appearing as I requested He had saved my bacon. Otherwise I would have been compelled to tell the doctor that yes *I have seen Jesus* and then what? Had Dr. Haynes noticed a smile creep across my face as I thought about God's sense of humour?

When I related this incident to Ron we shared a good laugh but he hoped in future sessions the doctor would not try to tamper with my faith.

~

In the meantime Ron and I had decided I should suspend my teaching job and try to work part-time pricing stock in the warehouse of the store he managed. We hoped I might get some satisfaction by working in a less demanding environment while my psychiatrist tried to assess my needs. But my symptoms grew more troublesome. Lower back pain, more intensive nausea and near fainting episodes had us very concerned. Ron urged me to take frequent breaks at work to rest.

The day came when Dr. Haynes announced he had arrived at a verdict. Once more he followed his pipe ritual. I wanted to snap with impatience while he knocked out the stale ashes and filled the barrel with new leaves. Only after taking several long draws did he swivel around to face me. His face gave no indication of the diagnosis he was about to convey.

"Mrs. Morgan, after interviewing you for the past few months I have arrived at a conclusion which will surprise you."

He waited for my response.

"Nothing you say will surprise me."

"You insist that something is very wrong with you." He cradled his pipe watching me.

"I don't know what to believe anymore." Maybe I was insane after all, I thought.

"It's no wonder." Dr. Haynes hesitated. "Mrs. Morgan, I'm afraid my colleagues have done you a great disservice."

What was he talking about? A disservice!

"What I'm saying is that I believe you."

"You do? " This psychiatrist believes me?

"I want to prepare you… for bad news."

I stared at him.

"I believe you are seriously ill."

I shook my head. No.

"I assure you Mrs. Morgan, you are quite sane. In fact you are to be commended for functioning so well given your degree of illness."

How was I supposed to grasp this new revelation — a complete reversal of all previous doctors' opinions? Should I rejoice? Or weep? Not crazy but seriously ill?

So, if I had been right all along then why had no one listened?

I had steeled myself to accept a diagnosis of mental illness — not this! Not serious illness… not after the consensus of professionals all these years! This could not be happening.

To underline his previous words Dr. Haynes stated, "Mrs. Morgan, I believe that you are critically ill."

"Critically ill!" The diagnosis had escalated to unreal proportions. A psychiatrist diagnosing a medical illness when the family doctors diagnosed me as psychosomatic?

"Your previous doctors missed some obvious signs in your basic bloodwork," he explained.

"So… they were careless."

Dr. Haynes nodded. "They wrote you off a long time ago… but now we need to focus on getting you well."

My turn to nod. "So what do we do next?"

"I am referring you to a kidney specialist in Greater Toronto asking for immediate attention. Their office will call you with an appointment date."

With this game-changing news I left Dr. Haynes' office... drowning in denial. I sat in my Valiant for a long time before driving back home.

~

chapter 5
Furry distraction, shocking outcome, loving promise

Commuters paced along the concrete platform. A businessman shifted his brief case to check his watch. What delayed the GO train today? A child pulled on his mother's sleeve, whining to be held.

Looking for some place to sit, I steered around a group of college girls with books propped in their arms. Wearily I slid into the *Plexiglas* cubicle with the fewest people.

The air was already warm for a May morning in a Toronto suburb. I pressed my fingers against my aching temples and tried to make sense of why today's trip to a kidney specialist was necessary. Fixing my gaze on someone's brown shoes, I let my mind track back to the previous week…

~

"Eek! Get that thing out of here!" I kicked at the six-week kitten wedged between my foot and the gas pedal. "Mark, grab that animal right now!" I shrieked. "I don't know how I let you kids talk me into this."

"Oh Mom," my nine-year-old son laughed, "We only picked Shelly up from the pound five minutes ago and already you're having a bird." Mark cupped the ball of fur in his hands, letting her tongue explore his face.

"Mark, my turn now!" Paul's chubby face framed in thick bifocals peered over the car seat. His hands groped for the new pet.

"Uh, uh," his brother teased. "She belongs to me."

From the back seat came a low howl. "M-o-m! Mark says the kitten is his. Give it to me, you dummy!" Paul pummelled Mark's head.

The car wheels squealed to a halt on the shoulder of the road. "Stop this nonsense right now!" I hissed. "Cool it, the both of you, or the thing goes back!"

Both boys knew they better not trifle with me. Young as they were, they sensed that something was wrong — something that had nothing to do with my discomfort around cats. After the bombshell from Dr. Haynes I had grown increasingly irritable. Nearly every day I wept with fatigue, wondering what final diagnosis lurked ahead.

Ron, however, was relieved that the psychiatrist had not written me off as 'psychosomatic'. Now we would get some answers about this mysterious illness that had disrupted our household.

"Sorry Mom," Mark sighed, handing the kitten to Paul whose eyes gleamed with triumph.

~

I roused myself from the daydream to see if the GO train was approaching. People still paced; the crowd multiplied. I returned to my thoughts.

The boys' kitten had joined our family a week ago providing them with a comforting distraction from the recent passing of their Grandpa Morgan and my unstable health. My own intolerance had evaporated as Shelly looked to all of us for food and affection.

When I came downstairs that morning to start breakfast, my spirits flopped at the sight of our kitten. Instead of pouncing on her dish of food Shelly stared listlessly at me, her head drooping against her shoebox.

Cradling her in my lap I drove to the veterinarian down the street. His diagnosis spelled trouble. Distemper, he said, was usually fatal. Even with antibiotics she only had a 20% chance of survival. I prayed that our boys' new pet would not die in the midst of everything else.

~

At the GO station the ground began to tremble. Dust swirled in little eddies, sucking bits of paper into its orbit. Shoulders rounded and arched forward to guard against the flailing wind and gathering roar of the advancing train. Commuters pushed toward the platform anticipating where the cars would stop.

Too weary to move, I remained seated behind the shelter until the train had shuddered to a full stop. I rubbed my lower back. For weeks it had ached like a bad tooth. Pain and nausea rippled in my groin.

Today... another specialist, this time in metro Toronto. Another blind alley and a waste of precious time. But the doctor's secretary judged differently.

When I returned from the vet, I called the kidney doctors' office to cancel my appointment, explaining that something more important had come up. Then I hung up. A few minutes later the phone rang. "Mrs Morgan," her voice sounded vaguely condescending. "I strongly urge you to keep your appointment with Dr. Bergen," She added, "It can't wait!"

I asked to reschedule for another day but the secretary used silence as leverage to cut through my delay tactics.

"Well, all right, but I can't make it on time." I glanced at the clock on the stove shelf. "I've already missed one train."

"Just come as soon as you can. I'll hold open an appointment for you."

I resisted hurrying. Instead, collecting a bowl of water and an eyedropper I showed Mark and Paul how to feed their pet. "Poor kitty," we lamented, stroking her nose.

~

"Mrs Morgan, hi!" A hand yanked me from my reverie. I looked up into the fresh face of a former student from our church youth group.

"Linda... it's been a long time."

"Come on, the train is here!" The perky young lady led the way joining the stampede for a seat. "Maybe I can find two seats," she called back.

I knew it was rude, but perky was the last thing I wanted. Shoving against the press of passengers I fled to another coach where I found a window seat.

In a stupor I watched the flash of suburbs and fields framed in the window while the train hurled itself from one sub-station to the next. With each stop new travellers boarded. All around me seats filled up. I huddled against the windowsill to discourage conversation and let the sweeping scenes soothe my frazzled mind.

Soot-laden factories and glimmering high rises. Slivers of sunshine glanced off the Toronto waterfront. An airplane, toy-like in the smog, seemed to melt into the CN Tower. A mile-high sign sponsored by a cereal company flashed the date, time and weather. May 26, 1982. 11:22 am. Sunny. Intermittent clouds...

Darkness leapt over our compartment as the train entered the city station tunnel. People spilled into the aisles grasping brief cases and bracing themselves for the stop. The train lurched and screeched before heaving its last long sigh.

Doors snapped open. As a unit the masses flowed from every doorway onto the platform, sweeping me along with the deafening current that rolled down the stairways and corridors and emptied into the mighty Union Station.

Dropping my arrival stub into one of the turnstile boxes, I shielded my eyes against the sudden intrusion of electric lights. My heart beat too fast. I fumbled toward a bench. After a few minutes the pounding let up. I proceeded to the long ramp descending into the subway station. A sleek noisy train shot from a tunnel and halted. The doors wheezed open allowing commuters only seconds to board before they closed with only the warning of a whistle blast.

Once again the train propelled itself into the ground.

Moments later our car emerged into the blinding daylight. The din of traffic made me recoil. I found shelter beside the graffiti-covered wall of a construction site where I checked the address scrunched in my pocket. Not much further now. Only one city block to the tall mud-brown building that housed the specialist's office.

After showing my OHIP health card to the secretary I sat down, resentful of wasting a beautiful spring day in a waiting room. The usual magazines filled a rack. I didn't bother with them. My mind flipped through a file of useless worry. Were the boys going to remember to feed their kitten at lunchtime? Would there be enough leftovers for supper?

Fifteen minutes passed since my arrival. Come on Doctor! What is keeping you? Let's get this session over with so I can go home and get on with life. Who was I kidding? Get on with life? First we needed answers. This could be the day.

A tall, distinguished man ushered me into his office, introducing himself as "Dr. Bergen". Unsmiling he asked, "Why do you think you've been sent to me?"

"Oh, I understand that recent tests have shown traces of kidney infection… but I'm sure it's gone by now." Shrugging, I looked past him at a photo of his young family. I wonder if he's a person who plays with his kids, I muttered inwardly.

He leaned forward obstructing my view of the picture. His eyes caught mine.

I wanted to look away. I knew what was coming next. He is going to tell me that there is nothing wrong with me… that all I need is a good shrink to fix my head. Ironically, I was discounting the psychiatrist's recent affirmation that I was perfectly sane.

His gaze refused to release me. Raising a brown folder he said, "This envelope contains your latest test results."

"Uh, huh…"

His eyes and tone reminded me of my rare visits to the principal's office when I was a kid. "They show me that there is a lot wrong with you!"

My breathing seemed to stall.

"There are microscopic particles of blood present in your urine… your fingers are cold to the touch… you seem to have undergone a personality change… and you demonstrate an inability to concentrate."

I waited for the rest.

"Your creatinine level is elevated. That is because your kidneys are likely working at less than 50% efficiency."

He read the question my raised eyebrow made.

"Meaning, Mrs. Morgan, that your body is loaded with poisons — probably has been for a long time."

The harshness seemed to leave his voice and expression. "You are a very sick woman."

Dumbly I followed Dr. Bergen's gesture to enter the exam room where his skilled hands investigated my glands, joints, and reflexes. "How are you feeling right now? Do you have any nausea or weakness? Any pain in your lower back or groin area?"

At that moment I could truthfully answer that I felt nothing. All the symptoms of pain and nausea that had plagued me for months and years receded in the face of this man's grave news. He was confirming the psychiatrist's pronouncement. Something really was seriously wrong.

"I want to hospitalize you right away."

"No! Please! First let me go home."

"Mrs. Morgan, it is urgent that you be hospitalized as soon as possible."

"Okay, but first give me time to go home and break the news to my husband in person."

Dear God, Ron will never believe this. They've given me the runaround for so long... but this time I know they are right. And yet I can't believe this! Someone has actually put his finger on my problem. This is real.

The doctor agreed to admit me in a week. His unexpected warmth unnerved me more than his initial crisp manner.

~

Barely seeing, I stumbled from his office and crossed over to St. Michael's Hospital to pick up a form from Admitting. As I left the maze of scrubbed hallways I passed a cloth banner embroidered with flowers and these words: *Bloom where you are planted.* The message meant nothing to me — yet I filed it away in case this was something God wanted me to remember.

As I joined the flow of sidewalk traffic outside the complex, my tears ran without restraint. For once I did not care that pedestrians watched my careful mask peeling away like poorly hung wallpaper.

After finding my way back to Union Station, I boarded the five o'clock train bound for the west end suburbs of Burlington and my family.

~

The week before my hospitalization skimmed by in a blur. Our kitten seemed to come around a bit and that cheered us up as we continued to pamper her. Ron and I decided we would wait until all medical investigation was completed before planning our future. I suppose we were not sure how to respond until all the evidence was in. Easier to hold out for a less dramatic diagnosis.

My close friend Helen asked if she could accompany me on the GO Train to St. Michael's Hospital. On that June morning full of bird songs she eagerly carried my suitcase because she wanted to spare my energy and share the experience with me. With typical generosity, Helen ignored her limited budget to buy an extravagant bouquet for my room from a flower vendor at Union Station.

At the end of two weeks of extensive testing and a kidney biopsy, Dr. Bergen met with Ron and myself to discuss the bottom line. He was forthright but kind. My condition had a name – end stage renal failure. My kidneys were both operating at about 20% efficiency. They were in the last stage of expiry and would shortly stop functioning altogether. I would soon require tri-weekly life-saving dialysis. Dr. Bergen hoped that with some care in my diet, such as salt restrictions, I could forestall dialysis for a few months. He emphasized that my childbearing years were over. My body could not support a new life.

In conclusion he gave a piece of surprising advice. He suggested I go home and give myself permission to be as sick as I felt: suspend the brave front for a while. He wanted me to realize the extent of this life-threatening illness by giving in at last to the symptoms.

News spread throughout our townhouse neighbourhood and our church family. Casseroles and home baked goods, notes and cards, glutted our refrigerator and our mailbox. Prayers were sent up on our behalf and hugs were delivered to our doorstep as people dropped by to support us. At first it was embarrassing. *All this fuss for what? This had to be a mistake — an overreaction.*

We just wanted to retreat and catch our breath. The definitive diagnosis we prayed for had finally arrived and it was far more serious than we imagined. We gave the news to our sons, however with as much optimism as we could muster, explaining that I had a kidney illness and doctors had a very effective treatment for it.

As well, during my last week in St. Michael's our sick kitten succumbed to her illness. Shelly had not been with us very long but she had provided a reprieve from serious matters — now that buffer was gone. It left me wondering if I too would go that way, but I kept that to myself. For the moment we didn't know how to feel, except numb.

~

The Saturday evening that followed the final diagnosis we tucked our youngsters into bed. Then my love, Ron, and I huddled close to each other on our soft living room carpet. Sipping our wine by candlelight we savoured the luxury of our intimacy before entering the roughest time of our lives.

We talked about our new reality; thus far we had only experienced the first throes of illness. Now that the phantom had a name and a treatment, Ron reasoned that we faced many weeks of separation as more hospitalizations became necessary. We really had no clue about how extensively kidney failure would alter our lives.

Lying in each other's arms, we clung to hope in the One who had brought us together and knew how to keep us safe through sickness and health.

"I love you, Elizabeth," my lover caressed my hair and my name. "You will see," he promised, "we will make it."

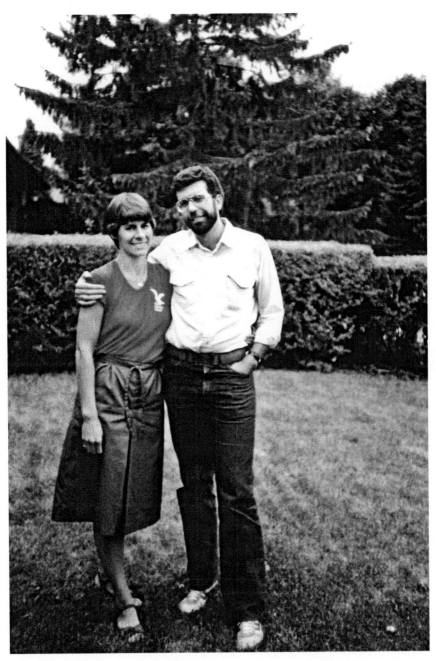

We reassure one another we will make it, Burlington

~

At first I followed Dr. Bergen's advice by allowing myself to give in to my illness. I often awoke with night sweats and terror that shook me with sickening dread. *What would become of us? Would I die?*

Ron urged me to make a train trip to Ottawa to visit old friends, Andrew and Hazel Penny. Five-year-old Paul and I made an adventure of it, packing several lunches for the overnight journey, riding the glass-domed car where we could see for miles and forgetting for a while about my condition. My solemn boy pressed close to me and I to him.

Andrew and Hazel took us under their wing, graciously insisting we use their master bedroom. Throughout the second night I vomited violently. My friend bathed me with warm water and with her shared grief. As morning broke she fed me a light breakfast, urging me to replenish my strength while she ensured Paul was cared for as well.

What must this have been like for Paul to see me so wretchedly ill? My friend likely explained to him that his mommy would get well soon and that Jesus would take care of us.

~

As I sat on the front step of our townhouse soaking in the sun I pondered how Jesus would do that — take care of us. My longing for assurance turned into a prayer. Would Jesus please come to me in a way that I could grasp? One of my teen Sunday School students told me the Lord had appeared to her mother during a difficult pregnancy. Lord, *I wish You would show Yourself to me that way, too.*

At night when everyone was asleep my fears often overtook me. Dreams reflected choking anxiety. When I awoke I would pray away the bad images and ask for better dreams.

A few weeks after my prayer I fell into a deep sleep that seemed different from any I had ever had. I dreamed that the boys and I were seated in our townhouse playing a board game, waiting for Ron to come home from work. He was working late and it was dark out. We had left the front room drapes open so we could see Daddy stride up the walk when he arrived.

While we waited a bright light filled our picture window. An image appeared in the distance, the shape of a man. He was approaching with lightening speed and yet moving very slowly at the same time — a strange sensation. Although I could not make out the features, I knew the face. It was the face of someone who loved us more than anyone. It was Jesus.

I grabbed my boys' hands and danced round and round. "I told you He was real! I told you He was coming!"

My boys laughed with me until we found ourselves caught up in the air, as our Lord came closer with arms stretched forward.

"I told you He was real!" I shouted to my neighbours who had ignored my pleas to listen.

When I awoke in the morning I knew that God had given the gift I asked for. He knew best. He had addressed my deepest desire, my greatest hope, since childhood: Jesus is coming again for those who will trust Him as Lord of their lives.

Yet what did this joyful dream have to do with the wretched reality we were currently facing?

It would take time to work that out, but for now God had reminded me that this world is only a temporary home; the real one awaits us in heaven.

Ultimately His purposes would be fulfilled through this illness and the stress laid on us as a family. Jesus is coming again, but for now I could trust Him to ground us in His reliable love.

~

chapter 6
Snuffed-out dream, new horizons, professional listener

My diagnosis delivered another kind of disappointing news. Although we had finally accumulated the money to buy a store, the Canadian Tire Corporate Head Office rejected our application when they learned of my prognosis. Since this was supposed to be a "mom and pop" venture, they did not want Ron to run it with the burden of a sick wife.

Ron's dream to acquire his own hardware franchise had been snuffed out. I was heartbroken for Ron. Guilt could have smothered any morale remaining after I realized my health had punctured his dream. But somehow I received assurance that God would open other doors for him. Ron was magnificent. He never placed a burden of guilt on me. When offered an executive position in the Toronto head office he turned it down, choosing rather to devote his energies to caring for us through our long-term crisis.

There must have been times when Ron struggled with anger at the unfairness of it all. If that was so he never let on. Ron's decision came from his commitment to put us first. I believe it also sprang from his commitment to listen to God's guidance — even when that meant suspending his own career advancement.

My husband's unselfish act inspired me to write a poem for him. As I spread a blank sheet on our kitchen table I asked the Lord to help me adequately express my deep respect and love for "this man, my mate." When Ron read it his tears told me all I needed to know. He asked if I would arrange to have it framed. While the composition to honour my hero came from my heart, I believe the Lord had directed the message.

My love
he makes me
feel so proud,
this year
he's come out
taller still.
In my eyes he is
a man among men
who dares to stand
and face the truth,
to speak it
when he must.

A man
who dares
to see beyond
the bluster
of a brittle
and unyielding heart,
that cries out
to be heard.

To me he is
a man among men
who never lets
a worthy dream
fall dead…

But rather
picks it up
and lets it
take new shape,
and his challenge
to every man
is, "don't allow
bitterness to overtake."

He's not too big
to hug his sons,
to say, "I'm sorry
and I love you."

Not too big
to wrap his gentleness
around his grieving mother.

Not too big
to bend his knee
before the sovereign Lord
alone.

To me he is
a man among men
who dares to love
supremely,
who would even
give up
a cherished dream
for those he loves the most.

There is a proverb –
describes him well,
"a man of understanding
walks straight."
how did I ever
gain such favour
to win this man
– my mate.

~

Not to be beaten down, Ron began a job search in the field of troubleshooting for the same company, Canadian Tire. Having earned an excellent track record in inventory control, Ron received several management offers from different provinces. He said it did not matter to him which job he accepted, so he asked which location I preferred. Ron said that since I was the one facing major illness, I ought to choose where I might fare best. Of all places — I chose Moose Jaw. I realized that my shaken spirit yearned for a return to the wide-open prairies of my childhood, a landscape that would relieve the sense of being closed in by uncontrollable circumstances.

Once we got used to idea of moving to another province we began to relish the adventure. Saskatchewan offered a slower pace of life far removed from the congestion of the Toronto suburbs. Leaving our family tree, home church, school, and friends became another matter. But we reasoned that our boys would adapt, and so would we. When my mother showed me a word of wisdom from a *Readers Digest* I felt emboldened about our decision. It said: *Man cannot discover new horizons until he leaves the shore.*

~

After saying our brave goodbyes to Ron's parents and my siblings and mom we pulled away from town with our *U-Haul* caravan of fellow adventurers — three vehicles carrying our foursome, good friend Helen, and several former employees who would help Ron to solve the management problems of the Moose Jaw store.

Before heading down the highway we pulled into the local service center for our fill up. A handsome man with a familiar hitch to his gait and a crooked smile greeted us.

"Dad! How did you know we would be here?"

His eyes twinkled. "Well, you know I have my spies. Besides I had to see my daughter and her family off one more time."

How my father loved to be on the giving end of a good surprise. Not one to expose sentimental feelings he never hinted at the underlying sadness of this farewell. Instead he anticipated the good times ahead for us.

When we finished our break, Dad followed us to the car. He held a parcel out to me. I don't remember what he said but I sensed the grief he felt for his daughter's uncertain future. Like the dad in that ballad who asks, "Where are you going my pretty one, pretty one?" was my father also wondering where this journey would take me?

Unwrapping the brown paper, I found a book called *The All Sufficient Christ*, a study guide on the book of Colossians. A book Dad chose just for me. For this journey into the unknown: to a new setting, a new set of battles relating to critical illness and survival. Through this gift my dad said all that a daughter ever needs to hear from her father's heart about his love, grief, and conviction that Christ is able to care for one's beloved children. The All Sufficient Christ would surely care for all of us.

Leaving "the shore" was wrenching but my heart was comforted and glad for a new adventure to embrace. We paused often for pit stops, meal breaks, and enjoyment of the changing countryside. At one stop we took advantage of the hotel pool, whirlpool and good dining.

Upon reaching the Saskatchewan border we all poured out of our vehicles. "Ee-haw," we hollered as we gathered to have our photo taken. The sight of endless wheat fields and smell unique to prairie earth made us giddy with joy. We were sure we had entered our promised land.

~

The boys enjoyed exploring Moose Jaw with us.

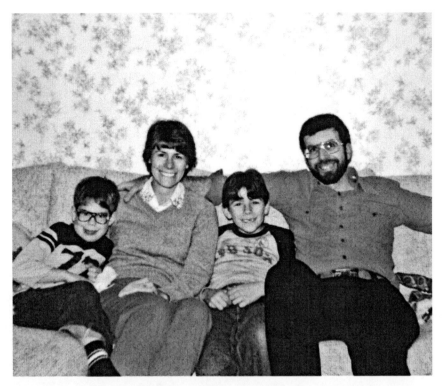

Enjoying our new horizons in Moose Jaw 1982

We bicycled up and down the wide prairie town streets where drivers took their sweet time. The boys tried out the spring-fed mineral pool downtown, and chased cheeky gophers popping in and out of their holes in nearby fields. We visited the three-story brick school they would be attending. We enrolled them in soccer and baseball, and found a church from which we hoped new friendships might spring.

~

For the first few months I think the adrenalin rush of a new setting masked my symptoms and awareness of the difficult road ahead. But as autumn leaves crumbled beneath our feet and snow followed soon after, the reality began to close in. I was growing thinner, paler and alarmingly yellow. Our patience with one another grew thin as well.

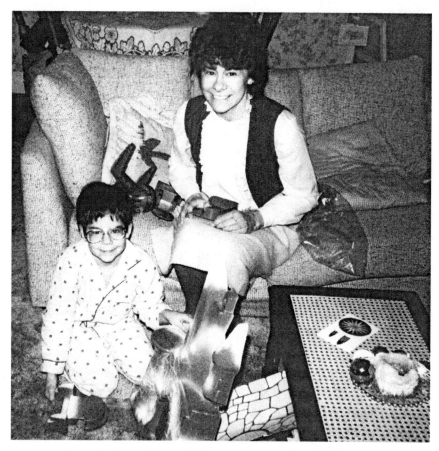

Turning yellow, puffy and worn out, Moose Jaw

That winter of '82 we began to face our monthly two-hour road trips for kidney assessment at Saskatoon's University Hospital with apprehension. On one such trip Ron seemed distant, not reaching for my hand to reassure me as he often did. What was he thinking about? I could not get inside his head and I felt volcanic.

"You don't care how I feel anymore!" I erupted.

"All I ever hear is how tired you are," Ron answered his voice as flat as the landscape.

His eyes followed the road ahead. "Well, frankly Liz, I'm tired too! Tired of your illness!"

There it was. The truth. He was tired of me. That is the message I heard, though not intended.

We watched the frozen prairies roll by while fear grasped us by the throat. We had never resorted to bickering or tearing each other down. What was going to happen to us? How would our fourteen-year marriage ever withstand the severe test thrust upon us?

~

On my next visit to "Dr. Rose", the kidney specialist, he told me the time for dialysis was imminent. He recommended I see a psychiatrist in my town to prepare me for the next stage. I welcomed the suggestion, knowing that a professional listener would help.

It turned out that the psychiatrist I was referred to was more qualified than most to help me cope with what was coming. This good man had actually been on dialysis for several years before receiving a kidney transplant. When he said he understood my fears I knew it was not empty reassurance. He forewarned me of some of the challenges I could expect to face: an unsightly arm for one thing, where needles would be inserted to deliver my blood to a cleansing filter and then return it to the same arm. He showed me his own scarred arm so that I had no illusions. He built up my confidence by expressing belief in my ability to face each day as it came, especially given my solid faith in God.

~

As I grew weaker and more nauseous, I felt motivated to attend a seminar held by an alternative health professional. After registering at the welcome table I turned to a friendly man near me and said, "I hope the guest speaker isn't boring."

He smiled, "I hope so, too."

I smothered a laugh when my neighbour strode up to the podium to introduce himself as the guest speaker we had come to hear. Thankfully for both of us he was anything but boring.

Ron and I decided to travel down to his alternative medicine clinic in Portland, Oregon. Perhaps his regimen of blood tests and natural products would delay the need for dialysis.

On our journey there we rented a seaside room for several nights at Canon Beach where we walked barefoot along the miles of sand bars. Ron believed in the philosophy that the best time to be happy is now. Now is what we had and he wanted to ensure that we did not waste time wishing we had enjoyed one another more. Sunsets over the water set the dunes on fire. Ron collected a bottle of sand and bought us a miniature sand castle so we would always have this memory for harder times.

~

chapter 7
Shocking revelation, mysterious kidnapping, answered prayer

Those harder times came too soon. Although the Portland Clinic staff was compassionate and friendly they could not reverse my kidney failure. In fact I became so ill we had to hurry home to see my own specialist.

Dr. Rose admitted me to the University Hospital in Saskatoon where I was given another kidney biopsy and surgery was performed on my left wrist to create a fistula. An artery and vein were sewn together to create a higher volume of blood in the finer surface veins where large needles would eventually be inserted for the procedure called hemodialysis.

However, first my doctor wanted to see how I would adapt to a less intrusive type of dialysis called peritoneal. This was supposed to be easier on the heart but I was one of those patients whose abdomen did not respond well to the bags of saline fluid dripping into my peritoneal cavity. Day after day I writhed in pain from the pressure that ballooned my stomach. Surely my body would soon adapt to the additional fluid.

~

This time was very hard on Ron. He could not bear to see me in pain; there was not a thing he could do to make it better.

So he went shopping. Not for himself but for me. Always ready to provide for me and to boost my morale, Ron surprised me with an attractive new outfit to hide the considerable tummy bulge on my otherwise slim frame caused by the litres of saline. As Ron helped me slip on my new clothes we overheard my dour roommate on the other side of my curtain whisper to her sister, "Edith, that girl is not going to make it."

Horrified at this pronouncement — maybe because they echoed our worst fears — Ron wanted to snap at my elderly roommate to 'shut up' and I wanted to sob. Instead my love led me into the hospital corridor for a stroll. "Hon, don't pay any attention to doomsday talk from negative people."

Ron assured me, and maybe himself too, that I would not always be in pain and that I would soon be well enough to return home. And then he kissed me goodbye. He needed to hurry back to our sons who were being cared for by caring neighbours. I dared not think about how much I missed my boys. Ron promised to bring them along on his next visit.

~

During one of my first hospitalizations I lay in my bed, too weary to care much about anyone else but myself. I watched as nurses about my age walked briskly by on their way to answer calls and do their duties. Long sigh. *I used to walk like that... was once pretty and young like them. I once enjoyed the strength of my youth and vitality... I will never be like that again.*

I tried to ignore the pleas of other patients. "Nurse! Nurse, help me!" And the moans of a man down the hall who was dying. A woman slowly paced the hallway, passing my doorway many times. She looked so very sad, yet peaceful. She must be the wife of the dying man. I overheard conversation that confirmed that. What hope could anyone give her! *O dear Lord, please help her through this. And her husband, please ease his suffering.*

I thought about my own family at home in Moose Jaw and how hard this must be for them. *Jesus, we need you. Please send us cheer. I sensed that I was dying along with that man.*

After some hours had passed, the lady stopped in front of my doorway and came to my bedside. She leaned close to me and whispered to me. "You love Jesus don't you?"

"How did you know that?" I could not believe how she knew that. There would have been no evidence to point to that fact.

"I know by your smile."

I didn't realize I was smiling.

She nodded. "It is Jesus smiling in you." And then she left as quietly as she had come.

My eyes blurred. How incredibly beautiful that Jesus could still shine through my misery... through a smile. And give comfort to someone else who loves Him. And then I remembered what my Sunday School teacher had revealed to me when I was eleven: *Your gift is your smile.*

~

One afternoon after gathering the energy to tidy up and get dressed, I overheard more from the sisters on the other side of my curtain. Ethel again whispered hoarsely, "Did you know that these young girls today like the one behind the curtain, shave their legs — can you imagine that? And they wear those new-fangled nylons with panties attached; pantyhose they are called. Can you imagine that, Esther? A person could get strangled in them things!"

Instead of feeling insulted I nearly laughed out loud and had to press my pillow against my mouth to stifle my snorts and giggles. What unexpected fun. Waiting I listened for more revelations.

Esther, the less ancient — but fashionable — sister with hair dyed red and impossibly high heels, managed to fake astonishment at my decadent ways. "It certainly is shocking."

More muffled sounds. What are they up to? Yikes. A highly decorated face peeked around my curtain. I smiled behind my pillow.

"Dear, we were wondering if you would like to share a little drink of something special I brought from home. "

"Oh no... thank you," I said wagging my hand, "I'm on a strict diet."

"Dear, you must try a little sip to cheer you up."

Okay, I would try just this once. The curtain was pulled back and a bottle was produced along with three glasses. Esther poured an amber liquid that she identified as a home recipe made with apricots. Just like the two prim so-called tee-totalling sisters of *The Waltons*, indulging their private vice, I thought. Won't Ron get a charge out of this story?

Clinking glasses together and lifting them high the old girls wished me good health. Later on as I drifted asleep I thought about how good God is to send relief in the form of humour, and a tender turn of heart.

~

After two weeks of witnessing my agonizing pain the doctor decided to end the experiment and send me home to rest and see my kids before the next medical intervention.

A few weeks later I returned. My stomach heaved as Ron and I rose early for my first day of hemodialysis. Kissing our boys goodbye we left before dawn for the long drive back to the Saskatoon Hospital. We prayed that I would be able to adapt; I had to, as no other options were available.

Round about Davidson the sun pulled up over the low horizon, taking our breath away: something lovely to remind us of God's abiding presence and care. Harder to remember His presence as we entered the hospital corridors in the basement to the treatment room where I was directed to a stretcher. A dialysis machine hovered nearby. Squeezing my eyes shut, I hoped I could block out my new reality. A male nurse lightly stroked my hand. A stinging odour assaulted my throat, the odour of disinfectant. Another nurse probed my left arm — the one designated as my dialysis arm.

"That looks like a good site," she said in low tones. She pressed again. Hesitated. Then she chirped, "Liz, are you ready? Okay, let's go for it!"

Swiftly steel met flesh. The big needle drove through to its bloody target.

I groaned. *Oh God, please help me!*

"We've got it in Liz. You're doing fine. Are you still in there?"

"I'm still here, " a small voice quavered.

"We're going to try the second needle now," said the chirpy voice.

Again a moist hand explored my left arm from wrist to elbow searching for a good site.

"Ready? Here we go!"

Another sharp thrust. More broken skin. And then it burrowed into a vein.

"Good girl, Liz! This part's done; you can come out now."

Wheels began to grind and groan. Carefully I opened my eyes. Turning my head to the left I saw blood-red streamers racing through miles of plastic tubing — my blood, miles of it — speeding out of my arm to be cleaned by this filtering apparatus and then allowed to rush back into the same arm.

Nausea ripped through me.

"Get me a kidney dish!" I yelled.

Sour bile spewed out, spilling over my sterile bedclothes and onto the polished floor. My stomach muscles rippled and retched, erupting more contents with volcanic force.

"Give her a shot of saline. Quick! Give her some gravol, too!" Raised voice, quick steps, more syringes, more pokes.

Gradually nausea subsided. I fell back onto my pillows, limp but still breathing.

I sighed, *thank you, Lord, I got through this part.* I'll get through the next three hours somehow... I drifted off, knowing that Ron sat nearby praying for me and for us as a couple and family.

~

Initiation day came and went. These three to four-hour dialysis treatments required us to drive to Saskatoon two mornings a week, and eventually three, always leaving before dawn.

A neighbour ensured our boys got up for school and took the lunches they had helped make the night before. The black ice and rutted roads of that prairie winter challenged Ron's considerable driving skills and nerves of steel. After each treatment I lay in the back of the car, often vomiting when I wasn't sleeping from exhaustion. Falling into bed after our long drives I did not have the strength to surface again until suppertime. The regimen took its toll on our morale, as did my numerous hospitalizations far from home.

~

For years I had kept a journal as a hobby and a way to reduce stress. With the shock of chronic illness my journal became my ally as I emptied my windstorm of thoughts onto its pages.

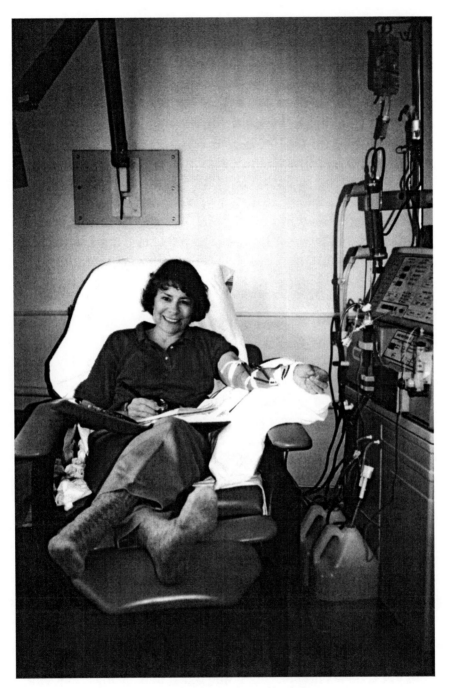

Journaling while on tri-weekly dialysis

Jacquie, the social worker assigned to me, stopped at my bedside one day and asked what I was writing. When I told her I was recording what it felt like to be sick and scared all the time she said, "Let me read it."

"No one reads my journals — they are intensely personal."

Jacquie persisted and since she had earned my trust by passionately advocating for me through my first days of hospitalization and peritoneal pain, I relented.

As she read she nodded, "How true! How true!" Her hoop earrings swayed in rhythm. At intervals she sighed.

When she finished reading the week's entries Jacquie let her bifocals dangle from their cord and leveled her eyes at me. I stared back, not knowing what comments to expect. Jacquie never withheld her opinion. My scribblings were raw; bleeding anger and self-pity. Not a pretty picture.

"Liz," she began, waving my green steno pad at me, "you have to share this with others!"

I folded my arms around my hospital gown and shook my head.

Jacquie would not be deterred. She leaned forward, "This week I have counseled at least six other patients on the heart and kidney ward." Pointing her red nails toward the hallway she continued, "Like you, they have gone through similar trauma. But they do not know how to describe their feelings."

Now she had my attention. Someone else hurts like me?

"If only they could read what you've written they would be so relieved to know that someone else feels the same kind of emotions: guilt for being a burden to their families, fear of further deterioration of health and… maybe death."

I could no longer see this imposing woman clearly. Why were we allowed to suffer so much? Life was too hard.

"Many people have doubts like you," Jacquie ploughed on, "but they are afraid to tell God how mad they are." She handed me a wad of Kleenex.

"I guess there's no point in hiding our rotten feelings from Him," I answered. "He knows we have them anyways. I think He's glad when we're still talking to Him, even if it is in anger."

Glancing at her watch, Jacquie stood up. "Please consider our conversation. I want you to think about sharing your experiences of the past few years." Turning at the doorway to look back at me she added, "In a book."

"A book?"

"I don't mean clinical data but rather the trauma of coping with chronic illness. Put that in a book."

Then she waved and was gone, leaving me with a great deal to think about. Perhaps some day I would write that book. For now I needed to get through this new way of living — in and out of hospitals.

~

When Ron came to take me home after one of my many hospitalizations, he had a serious one-on-one conference with my kidney specialist. Ron insisted on the bottom line. The news was sobering.

Dr. Rose advised my husband that I only had about a year to live.

Ron asked, "What will it take to help my wife recover? Tell me, and I'll do it… anything to give her more time. "

The doctor said this might be possible if I did nothing else but look after myself. The care of our sons and our household — groceries, meals, laundry — had to be left in Ron's hands.

I knew nothing about the specialist's shocking revelation of my short life expectancy. Ron revealed only what he felt was necessary information: the fact that we would have to restructure our workload so that I could be freed up to recover.

When we arrived home from Saskatoon Ron strode into our kitchen. "First thing I'm going to do," he announced, flinging open all the cupboard doors, "is rearrange your dishes."

I winced; Ron used to be a professional merchandiser. Keeping the contents of my cupboards orderly had never been my strength but I had embraced the kitchen as my domain. Although he must have been tempted, my husband had never before intruded upon my sacred territory.

Seating myself at the kitchen table I steeled myself for this changing of roles, another letting go of how things used to be. Calm on the outside, I held my breath.

After Ron pulled down our everyday dishes and dry goods onto the counter, he moved to the better dishes. I grimaced as my husband tried to make sense of my teacups piled in teetering pyramids. The tension mounted; I could smell a storm coming on.

In a flash all attempts to control emotion let go as Ron began to hurl china cups across the room, their fragile beauty smashing into tiny bits all around us. I recoiled. These pieces were my identity. The china cups, the kitchen — they symbolized my capabilities as a homemaker who had provided a refuge for my husband and children, a place of hospitality for our friends and guests.

The moment of truth had arrived; I had ceased to be useful and I wanted to run. Yet, more than my own dignity seemed at stake. I needed to stay and witness Ron's anger, to enter into his trauma as well as my own. His dreams had shattered too. My love was hurting too. Far more than I knew.

When the gale had subsided I retreated to our bedroom where I allowed grief to roll over me like a soft rain. After a while Ron entered the room and sat on the bed beside me. He cradled me in his sturdy arms. I felt his tears on my neck.

In this deeply sad moment we acknowledged our mutual pain and reinforced love's enduring promise: 'We will make it, you will see.'

~

"Hon, from now on we've got to keep current with what's happening," Ron said as he stroked my arm. "It's important for you to tell me what's on your mind." He wanted to understand my fears so that we could address them. But Ron rightly judged that it was not helpful to reveal the scary probability that I was dying. His goal was to focus our minds on living today.

To make sure neither of us let things slide, we scheduled weekly talk sessions at our kitchen table. We identified the problems created by my limitations. Brainstorming helped us find solutions concerning my personal care, household maintenance, and discipline along with emotional support for our boys. These conversations led to better utilization of everyone's time.

~

"Come on guys, let's make tracks!" Ron roused our sons from their sleepy daydreaming while they toyed with their cereal. "You've got chores to finish before you head for school."

Our chubby six-year-old peered through his bifocals to review the oversized chart on the porch door. In his foghorn voice Paul read the jobs allocated to him during our last family conference. "Paul: Take your boots off. Set the table. Dust all rooms."

His father dropped a load of laundry into the basement washer, while ten-year-old Mark struggled to change the beds. He checked the rest of his list, which included our new pet dog. "Take Skimmer out. Feed her. Thaw out supper. Clean the bathrooms."

Since the boys' attempts at cleaning washrooms, vacuuming and dusting eventually caused me undue stress — I wanted to clean after them — Ron eventually hired a housekeeper; an elderly man of seventy-four who used to keep house for his ailing wife and loved to make our place shine. While Bill cleaned I would attend a women's coffee hour feeling a little guilty for indulging such a luxury. But Ron reassured me this social outlet was an important expenditure of my energy; housework was not.

Ron and I agreed I would focus my limited energy on two responsibilities: care for myself and time for our sons. We studied all the implications of self-care. They included strict adherence to a daily regimen of diet and fluid restrictions, medications and rest. Meticulous grooming was also factored in. On those days when life seemed least appealing to me, fussing with makeup, hair and an attractive outfit proved a valuable means to bolster my morale. It also gave my family a lift. None of us could afford to bury ourselves in self-pity.

In order to avoid episodes of nauseous weepy exhaustion, I learned to pace my activities. This meant examining and reorganizing my priorities.

Numerous friendships always placed high on my must-do list, but now I needed to reserve my energy for my family. By surrendering my weary body to three-hour daily afternoon naps, I recovered sufficient strength to join the boys for evening activities. We discussed their school happenings while making popcorn, playing a game of Junior Scrabble or reading a story together.

Sometimes discipline posed a problem when the boys' arguments wore me down. We devised an escape measure. If I couldn't resolve the issue with them, I instructed Mark and Paul to call their dad at work. After a telephone conference our youngsters usually settled down. Since the store Ron managed was just a convenient block down the street he would sometimes have our boys come over for a coke and pep talk.

~

"Love can perish when there is no time for romantic activity."

Ron and I agreed with this quote by family doctor and author, Dr. James Dobson. We knew that even though we were committed to one another, we could not afford to take our love for granted. Ron had consistently gone out of his way to demonstrate his care for me, arranging time for the two of us, and leaving love notes on my pillow or breakfast tray.

But, time after time while hospitalized, I met fellow patients whose spouses had left them. I heard stories of how their mates could not bear the day-in and day-out drudgery of illness and the washed-up dreams. These stories picked away at me; would our solid marriage fall by the wayside as well? I inwardly questioned how my husband could want to see this through when there was always another health issue to address. It had to wear away at his morale and endurance. But I failed to discuss these fears with Ron — he had enough to worry about.

Irrationally and privately, I began to grieve for what I perceived as our fading love story. I lay awake shaking with fear of dying before my natural time or living a shadow of my former self. I feared for our children's wellbeing. I dreaded becoming an unbearable burden to my long-suffering husband.

Worse, I began to consider that my husband and children would be better off if I did not survive. I began to wish my illness would overtake me. Then my family could start over again with a healthy spouse and mother. These were among my darkest moments, fed by collapsing health, self-rejection, and a body full of poisons and constantly shifting electrolytes.

Not only was the warfare physical and emotional in nature, but spiritual as well. I remembered the teaching of God's Word that says our struggle is not only against flesh and blood but against the dark forces of evil. Satan — the enemy of our souls — wanted to undermine my trust in God and our family unity by feeding me black thoughts; lies about my worth to my husband and children.

~

These satanic lies sabotaged my mind until it all came to a head.

As I sat on the side of our bed I thought about how much I wanted to let go of all restraint and go mad. What would happen if I did let go?

A wretched sound erupted from the pit of my being. Gathering in momentum the pain within me howled like a trapped animal. God help me, I wanted relief. Somebody, please take the torment away!

Ron came running. What was wrong? What was this all about? I'm sure my eyes looked dead. How frightening for my protector who held me until I fell silent. Then he led me onto the back porch steps where we listened to summer crickets and waited for reason to return.

I let the poisonous thoughts spill, exposing my skewed beliefs that others could do a better job of replacing me as the boys' mother and imagining that Ron no longer wanted me in his life. Terror had gnawed away my confidence as a woman; I did not believe I was worthy of being loved as a wife or a mother.

Ron reassured me. We would try to find ways to give me a more active role in our boys' lives. As for the part about fearing our love story was over, Ron promised me it was still alive. Panic and despair had blinded me to the daily evidence that my husband was always a man who kept his promises.

Ron stated that leaving me was never a consideration. We were in this together. To drive home his point he reminded me about the time some fifteen years earlier when the Lord came quietly to him in his car and revealed to Ron that I was the one he was meant to marry. We were a team — put together by God — for the long haul. My fears were only nightmares; my reality was our solid love for one another.

"Focus on your reality," he urged.

~

Since weekly dates had been always been a part of our planning to keep the romantic fires burning, we planned a regular mid-week breakfast rendezvous at the local café with the hope that I could manage this. Often my head felt so heavy I wanted to slump onto the table and doze. But since my husband loved me enough to make the effort, so would I. He had the faith to believe that our efforts would pay off. My cooperation was needed.

Gradually my tri-weekly dialysis regimen began to clear the poisons more efficiently and I grew more alert. No doubt much energy had been wasted in keeping silent about my worst fears. When the volcano in me had finally exploded, the poisons of my mind found release. Although I felt great shame for not being strong enough, I held onto my God who would make a pathway through the rubble. I knew that Ron held onto Him too.

~

While I took my medications Ron breezed into the kitchen and kissed my head, "Morning, Hon."

He smiled playfully, "What would you say if we change our Tuesday breakfast date to a lunch outing today? Do you think you would be up to that?"

"Sure," I nodded, gulping down the last pill. "Why not? We can give it a try."

Excitement rose in me as I carefully dressed in a new pair of casual slacks and red-striped top Ron had recently bought for me. This was beginning to feel like an adventure.

When Ron came back for me at noon we drove downtown and stopped at a sub shop. After choosing our subs Ron informed me that we were not going to waste this beautiful afternoon eating inside. Hmm, where was he taking me? Although Moose Jaw had a few little parks, Ron drove to the edge of town and parked our car near an unlikely site, the town creek.

The creek area, Ron told me, had been renovated to make it more inviting to visitors. When he reached into the trunk to retrieve our sandwiches out came a big wicker basket, as well.

My spirit sparkled. Wow, a romantic date! Arm in arm we strolled until we found a park bench. Hikers passing by on the new board-walk smiled approvingly as we sipped wine from our goblets and I held a lovely silk rose.

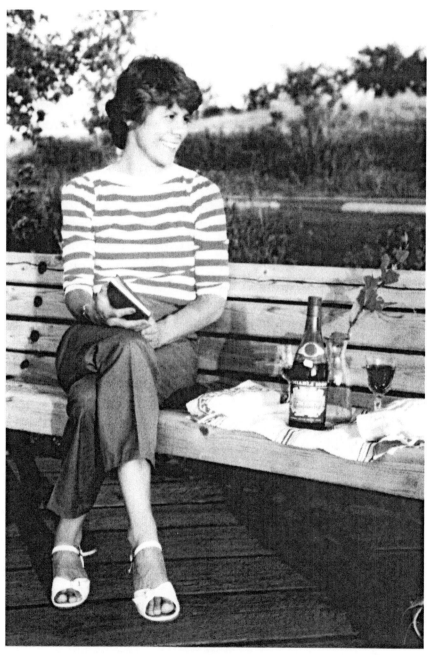

Ron whisks me away for a wine and sub picnic, Moose Jaw 1983

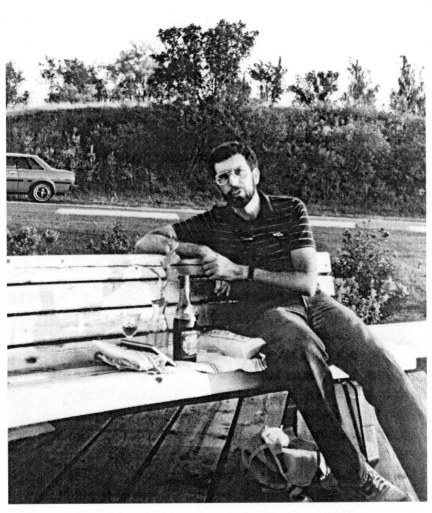

Ron enjoys surprising me with a romantic picnic

To top it off, Ron presented me with a red velvet-bound booklet of love poems. Even better, he paused to read one to me. 'My true-love hath my heart, and I have his… there was never a better bargain driven, my true-love hath my heart, and I have his.'

~

After completing my morning shower and grooming ritual I took time to journal in a cozy corner of our living room. So nice not to have to get up early for dialysis since my appointments were Mondays, Wednesdays and Fridays. I wrote out a prayer of thanksgiving as I remembered the amusing events of our recent family outing to Lethbridge Park where we played and picnicked together. Paul had us in stitches imitating his older brother trying to look cool for the young ladies tripping by.

Ah, it was so peaceful I could hear every hum of the refrigerator and creak of the floorboards.

The boys had shuffled to school and Ron had walked to work, so I was surprised when I heard his voice.

"Did you forget something?"

"Sorry to interrupt you, Hon… I think I left some paperwork in my dresser. Don't let me disturb you."

When Ron finished rummaging, he asked if he could take me for a drive and lunch at an upscale hotel restaurant on the edge of town. Oh sure, I was game.

"I'll be back in an hour."

A short time before his return for me I rechecked myself in the mirror. A few stray hairs had been missed while curling my hair earlier. But when I opened my cupboard I was mystified. *I was sure I left the curling iron here… must have put it elsewhere. Not in my top dresser drawer either. Hmm, this is driving me crazy!*

The porch door slammed. "You ready to go?"

Oh dear, I sighed, glancing back in the mirror. It would have to do; Ron would never notice if my hair was not perfect. But where did that curling iron go?

~

"You look lovely as always," my date said to me as we ate our gourmet meal and talked about how enjoyable it was to be together like this.

When we were leaving the hotel lobby Ron steered me toward the elevator. "Remember I told you about my Ontario business friend who is staying here? I would like you to meet him."

I thought how nice it would be to see a face from our former hometown. We knocked at his suite door but he didn't answer. Ron reached into his pocket and brought out a key.

"What are you doing?" I asked as he slid the key into the keyhole and turned it.

Ron turned to me with a silly grin. "Why don't you see for yourself," he said guiding me through the doorway.

I stood thunderstruck. On a coffee table stood a vase of roses, candles, and a white cake. On the bed lay one of my silky nightgowns, and on the dresser my swimsuit, underthings, toiletries — and my curling iron.

"What? How? When? Wow!" I beamed at Ron who was enjoying my utter delight at his surprise.

"You've just been kidnapped!" he announced.

Ron explained that when he had returned to find his 'paperwork' he was actually gathering up all my stuff hoping he could smuggle it out without raising my suspicions. I had conveniently been preoccupied with my writing. Ron anticipated everything I would need for an overnight stay right down to my medications and of course, supervision for our boys with their beloved sitter and friend, Carol.

In the evening after Ron and I shared a candlelight dinner, Carol brought our boys over for a pool party and cake celebration.

After hugging our clan goodbye, we fell exhausted into bed. Holding me in his arms my sweetheart whispered, "I love you Elizabeth and I never want to take you for granted."

I purred like a cat warmed by the sun.

~

"Hey Mom," my youngest called to me when he came home from school. "Our school is going to have a Monster House set up in the gym for Halloween night!"

Paul sounded very enthusiastic about this prospect. He explained further, "We have been asked to bring something creepy to touch in the dark."

"What creepy things do you have in mind?"

"Oh, stuff like slippery cold noodles or raw hamburger or plastic spiders or… "

"What else?"

"Well, I told the teacher I would like to donate your arm — that is something really creepy to touch!"

I looked at my dialysis arm with the newly acquired bulging purple veins and laughed. "You're right that would be very creepy."

Who would have guessed that I could ever learn to laugh at my unsightly arm! My sons' forthrightness and the curious stares from strangers and friends alike helped me to accept my left arm as a part of my reality and use it as a teaching tool. Whenever I had the opportunity, especially with kids, I liked to explain the purpose of my bulging vessels. They would listen with fascination and when they touched my fistula — the place where an artery and vein were surgically joined — they could feel and listen to the buzzing of that area, called "a bruit" or "a thrill."

I never did donate my arm for Halloween but Paul's idea gave us something to laugh about. Actually, he said my arm never did creep him out but his friends did ask questions that led to some fun discussions.

~

As I waited for Ron to drive me to the local bus station I heard Mark and Paul stop in front of our bedroom door.

Tap, tap.

"Come in," Ron called, raising his head from his kneeling position beside our bed.

98

"Dad, I've finished letting Skimmer outside, fed her and laid the plates out for supper," Paul said.

"And you, Mark?"

"Ya, Dad. I cleaned the bathroom and am thawing the casserole in the fridge."

"Good job, guys. I love you lots. Have a good day at school." Ron embraced them.

I thought how wonderful that our sons had a visual of faith at work as they observed their father's daily habit of kneeling to commit all of us to the Father's care.

At the station Ron held me close. "You'll do great, my love," he whispered into my hair. "Today is another day to keep you well."

The tri-weekly bus ride to Regina became my new routine after Dr. Rose decided I had stabilized sufficiently to transfer to a dialysis unit closer to home — an hour's ride rather than two and a half hours. This left more time for Ron with the boys since the bus ride was relatively short.

Looking out my tinted window, I watched the crisp blue sky pushing down against the frozen fields flattening them into one enormous sugar-dusted pancake. "A god-forsaken land... those damned prairies," I had heard one old timer say. But for me, a city girl fresh from the clutter of Toronto suburbs, the prairies of my childhood gave solace.

They soothed the panic ripping through me, the panic that often soaked my bedclothes when I would awake in the night and remember that these life changes were real.

The desolate beauty wrapped around my bus seemed to whisper that sometimes it was okay to be sad and weep for my once vital young body and mind. Chronic illness was still taking its toll on me. It felt like a big deal to get through one day with a measure of faith and humour.

Rummaging through my tote bag I retrieved a green steno pad and pen. I began to write out my despair: *Lord how I fight it — this daily burden of fatigue, nausea and more fatigue. At times I feel abandoned by You. And bitter beyond belief...*

What was that? I paused to listen. The sounds of a mouth organ quivered in the stale air of the Greyhound. Then nothing. Hmm, I must be hallucinating.

I resumed my complaints. *God, what are You trying to do to me? I can't bear this regimen of dialysis much longer. It's not fair. Why have You allowed this to happen to us? We were a happy family once. When will I be well enough to go for a transplant? Will I ever be normal again? I can't stand to witness all those sick yellow people at dialysis — yellow like me. My heart breaks for all of us. Wish I could die and get this over with...*

"Amazing grace how sweet the sound..."

There it was again! Now I swore I could hear a mouth organ.

Like an ostrich I lifted my head from my hiding place and scanned the aisle. There he was! Sitting kitty corner from me. Eyes danced in his corrugated face, his ancient hands and mouth caressed the instrument. Preoccupied in pleasure he continued as though making music on a bus wasn't the least bit unorthodox.

"That saved a wretch like me. I once was lost but now am found, was blind but now I see."

Tears trickled down to my smiling lips. I wasn't being forsaken after all. Instead of scolding me for questioning His input in my altered life He simply reminded me that His grace is changeless, still as amazing as ever.

~

"Liz, I think you are ready for a transplant," said Dr. Rose, who noted that dialysis was a temporary means for survival and that a graft would free me from that rigorous regime. He also warned us of the risks involved in transplantation, such as rejection. We appreciated his honest communication with us and trusted his judgement.

Dr. Rose suggested that I do two things: put myself on the recipient list for a cadaver kidney, and also approach my family tree to see if anyone was willing to be tested as a prospective donor. The chance of a graft's success was multiplied when related living donors were involved. Since I had six siblings there might be someone who matched my blood type.

Tests revealed that the sibling with the same blood type and closest match in several categories was my brother Ken, who lived in Zambia, Africa with his wife and children. Preliminary testing in South Africa indicated that the match was not ideal, but plausible. We were thrilled that Ken might be my donor since he had played an instrumental role in how Ron and I met. (Though Ken had warned Ron sixteen years earlier that I was "religious", he eventually became an overseas missionary!) And when he married Cathy, our close bond extended to her as well.

Two weeks before they were due to arrive at our place a call came from Dr. Rose.

"We think we have a cadaver kidney for you that could be a match. What would you like to do? Wait for your brother or see if this one will work?"

If this cadaver was a match we preferred to go for it and spare Ken the loss of his healthy kidney. Excitement mounted in us as we rushed up to Saskatoon for the final testing that would verify whether this organ would become my new lease on life. We talked about how it will be when I have a working kidney and no longer need to schedule dialysis runs.

Dr. Rose said the results had yielded positive outcomes; by morning I would be going to surgery. His grin told us he shared our excitement. Ron kissed me goodnight before spending the night in a nearby motel while I tried to sleep before the big event. But it was hard to do when our lives were about to take a new turn.

A nurse nudged me from my drifting thoughts. She wanted to know how many blood transfusions I had received since I started dialysis and had I ever had antibodies in my blood. I had required frequent transfusions to top up my anemic blood but I wasn't aware of any antibodies. Was that a problem? She said it was part of the routine of questions they need to cover when doing a transplant workup and urged me to rest up.

An hour or so later Dr. Rose stood at my bedside. He looked at my enquiring face and then he looked away. Without warning he hit his hand against the wall. What was this about? Did I see tears in his eyes?

"Liz, you have developed antibodies from your last blood transfusion. Rare antibodies." He explained that they would cause rejection. "We cannot give you this kidney."

For that moment I was more touched by my doctor's show of emotion than by the hard news. This guy really cares about his patients. What a rare gift of compassion!

In the morning Dr. Rose had more difficult news for Ron and me. He warned us that Ken may not have my newly acquired antibodies and we should be prepared for that disappointment. Only further testing upon Ken's arrival would clarify that matter.

Maybe God was testing our faith to see how far we were willing to trust Him.

~

Ron cautioned me not to get my hopes too high. But it was too late. My emotions were soaring. Surely I was not meant to live a life on dialysis indefinitely. For months we had been advancing toward this moment…

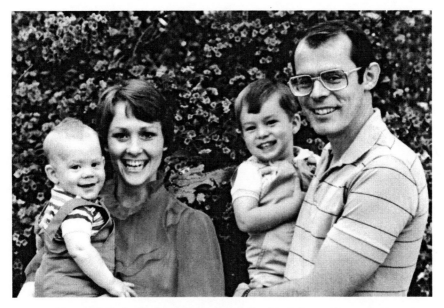

Ken and Cathy fly from Zambia to offer his kidney, Moose Jaw

Ken received the last round of tests at the University of Saskatoon. The day of decision had arrived. My kidney specialist would be calling with the final verdict. As we pulled out of the driveway, Ken and Cathy waved goodbye from our porch.

"I'm glad you came up with the idea to go away for the day," I said to Ron, inhaling the stinging February air and rubbing my fingers to keep warm.

Every farmer's field looked identical; a frosty plate of snow with stray stalks of yellow weeds thrust toward the ghostly sky. Fear alternated in us along with hope for what the day might produce.

"I thought it would be good for you to have a change of routine today," my love answered, reaching over to stroke my hair.

"Our friend in Estevan sounded really pleased to hear we were driving down for a visit, didn't she?"

"You know you have a lot of people rooting for you, my Elizabeth."

I smiled. Yes, I knew that. Many people from our former church in Ontario had not forgotten us. They were praying for us, along with those in our family tree and the few new acquaintances in our town.

Yet an uneasy feeling gnawed at me. What if Ken and Cathy had flown to Canada for nothing? Would my recently acquired antibodies conflict with those my brother had? Possibly. But God was still in the business of miracles — and we needed one.

After tea with our friend we drove home in the descending dusk. Circles of light from the porch and kitchen window welcomed us back. While Ron parked the car, I hurried up the steps and shoved open the side door. Blinded at first by the sudden glare in the kitchen, I could not define their faces. But I could feel the hush.

"Well? Did Dr. Rose call?" I blurted too loudly.

Slumping his back against the counter, Ken crossed his arms around himself. I searched his face for that telltale, crooked grin he gets when he is pleased. He stared at the floor.

"It's no go," he murmured.

Cathy rushed towards me, wrapped herself around me like a blanket and wept. I leaned against her.

After a while she held me at arm's length, looked into my eyes and whispered, "We wanted so much to help you."

My heart swelled with comprehension of their great love for us.

~

That night our two families crowded into the tight space surrounding our kitchen table. Even our wild youngsters seemed subdued, sensing the mood of the adults. Serving plates were heaped with good things Ken and Cathy had worked all afternoon to prepare: fried chicken, baked potatoes and parsley carrots.

We joined hands to ask a blessing upon our gathering and meal.

In his powerful bass voice, Ron began the round-robin prayer. "Dear Lord, we thank You for answered prayer today…"

My eyes darted toward my husband's bowed head. He's got to be kidding! Answered prayer? I wanted to kick him.

But my love continued his prayer of thanksgiving for God's care over us. Ron's words came from a heart that chose to trust that God had a better plan in mind for all of us.

Whether I wanted to accept it or not the day's results were answered prayer. We had asked God for a match and He had given His answer: No, my children — not today.

Closing my eyes again, I bowed my head while hot tears surrendered to my Father in heaven who knows best.

Yes Lord... thank You... for answered prayer.

On either side of me hands gripped mine. We were not left without comfort.

~

After the news that Ken could not be my donor, I returned to the hospital in Saskatoon where my specialist gave me more stinging facts.

The odds of my body accepting a transplanted kidney were one out of ten. He reminded me about the rare antibodies I developed from frequent blood transfusions. Meaning it would take a long time to find a kidney compatible to mine, cadaver or living donor.

"We are probably looking at a five-year wait."

After Dr. Rose left the hospital room, I wept into my pillow.

Five years on that demanding machine! How would I ever endure it? The few months already spent on dialysis were a living nightmare for me. Every time I walked along the corridor toward the dialysis room I felt overpowered by the odour of formalin, a powerful disinfecting agent. Waves of nausea had become my life.

Whenever the two darning-sized needles were inserted into my fistula arm I cringed. The nurses kept missing the narrow underdeveloped vessels. Squeezing my eyes shut I wanted to scream at them: STOP gouging, STOP digging! Sometimes after a second or third probe a nurse would call for another nurse or doctor to give it a try. The sight of my own blood racing through the bloodlines had me gagging and yelling for a kidney basin.

"Five more years of this!" I sobbed pounding my pillow. "I can't take this! It's not fair, it's not fair."

For years I had been misdiagnosed and now this. The medical profession had failed me. God had failed me.

~

In silence my questions toppled over each other…

Lord, what are You trying to tell me? Am I supposed to exist on a machine for the rest of my life? How many years have I left? This isn't supposed to happen to young mothers and wives. My husband and I — we need each other. My boys — this is too hard for them. It's not fair. I've tried to trust You all of my life. And now this.

The lashing torrent of accusations and objections ran dry.

I rolled onto my side and stared into the blackness. Alone. I'm so alone.

The hospital was over two hours from my home. There would be no visitors until the weekend. I didn't want to alarm Ron with a late night call to tell him the heartbreaking news. Only my doctor and I knew. And God.

I have no other hope but in You, Lord. I will lie here and wait until You speak.

My small white clock ticked steadily. And I waited.

Beyond my heavy closed door I heard the muffled laughter of night nurses at their station. Nothing more than that distant sound.

An hour passed. I don't know if I actually believed that God would answer me that night. I did not sense His Presence as I often had in previous crises. What did I wait for? An audible voice? No. I only waited for a sane thought to penetrate the dead shell of my mind.

Tick, tick, tick. Another hour passed. The formless black held my eyes captive as I huddled under the stiff cool sheets.

"Say, 'The Lord is my Shepherd, I shall not want.' "

Slowly I raised my head. *Who said that?*

There was no one there. No one that I could see. The words had seemed to come from my bedside. I strained to listen.

Then it occurred to me. What I heard was just a thought in my head. But… wasn't that what I was waiting for? A rational thought to break the deadlock?

For the first time in hours I began to speak audibly. Hesitatingly, the words I knew so well from childhood came forward. "The Lord… is my shepherd… I shall not want."

"Say it again."

There it was again — that gentle command.

I opened my mouth to form the familiar words once more, only this time with greater conviction. "The Lord is my donor, I shall not want."

Oh Liz, you know that's not how it goes. I laughed at my blunder. Donor? Where did that word come from?

The blunder was not of my own doing. Suddenly I knew that the Lord was having a conversation with me using my mind as His vehicle — the way He often does when we are serious about hearing His answers.

He was trying to penetrate my grief and at last I was getting the message. The Lord would be my donor. I was not at the mercy of human factors. Even though my future looked unbearable I didn't need to panic. He was raising my sights to see beyond the apparent realities. In due time the Creator of my body would provide the kidney I needed.

~

It was amazing to see the progress I had made since by my first days of dialysis. I was able to sit up and watch the whole procedure. The sight of my own blood speeding through the lines no longer made me ill. On one such day my nurse for that morning unsheathed the needle she was about to insert in me. Then she said, "Will you hold this for me a minute; I forgot something."

When she returned she leaned close and whispered, "See that couple over there?"

Yes, I had met them in the lobby.

"Well they own a farm and need to get back to it so they want to learn home dialysis but she is scared to needle her husband. So… here's what I want you to do." The nurse looked me in the eyes, " I told her that you are going to put in your own needles today for the first time and then she will see how easy it is."

I was flabbergasted. I looked over at the couple. The woman smiled expectantly. *Oh brother, what a trick!*

Of course I wanted to cheer them on so before I knew it I was following my nurse's confident instructions on how to insert the needle. Although I felt fearful as everything about the pain, she urged me to focus on technique instead.

As I guided the point into my vein it broke through my dry tough skin and glided into place like butter. Like butter. Bingo! It was in and I hadn't even noticed the pain.

Thereafter I was put in charge of my own needling; a good way to be more in control of my healthcare. Furthermore, that couple learned the procedure and went home to their farm.

~

Since I had made significant progress, my dialysis team and specialist suggested that home dialysis was possible for us too, if we learned how to do the whole procedure ourselves. That way I could be spared the stress of travel time and expense to the health care system. We decided to give it a shot. Our reliable friend Carol looked after our boys while Ron and I trained in St. Paul's Hospital in Saskatoon. I stayed in residence while Ron commuted three times a week.

Ron's role was to set up the machine and help me get hooked up to the bloodlines. I could insert my own needles, but Ron needed to learn this part as well. He caught on to the technical side of set-up and needling but the emotional component became a sore spot between us. With each solo dialysis run our tension festered.

Why were we snapping at one another? Was I not trusting that my husband could take care of me? We both knew so many things could go wrong. Too much seemed to ride on us and this experiment. If we could not "do" this I would have to keep on travelling and be away from home three times a week.

Ron finally admitted he resented the idea of home dialysis. It took more of his free time away, time already stretched thin. And it added more pressure on him. It threw off the balance of responsibilities he'd already taken on at home to free me up to devote my energy to the boys and him.

We asked God to guide us in deciding whether to finish training.

After Ron completed his part of the training he returned to the boys and business in Moose Jaw while I remained behind in Saskatoon to learn my parts. I had trouble remembering every step and I was homesick, not sure I wanted to continue with training we might never use.

The clincher came when Ron called from home.

"Liz, I think you should come home for a week."

"Why? What's wrong?"

"Paul is sobbing with loneliness for you."

That did it for me. We needed to rethink our options and lay our cards on the table. When crises arose cool heads were needed and this was the one thing Ron admitted he could not be cool about. "Not where you're involved, My Love. I hate being responsible for you; if anything went wrong and I hurt you... "

There were other reasons that made the idea of home dialysis unpalatable for us. We agreed it was too emotionally hard on us as a family to have the machine at home as a constant reminder of illness. There would never be any escape from the anguish and strain on our relationship and family life.

Our conclusion was unanimous. We needed to separate home and dialysis. Tri-weekly commutes to a clinic would have to remain a way of life for us.

For us this was the right decision.

~

On one of my non-dialysis days Paul volunteered a secret he had carried around for several years.

Sitting on a kitchen stool I started a stew for supper when Paul wandered in through the back door. A blast of chilly air followed closely behind. Kicking off his snowy boots he dropped his down jacket over them and dragged a chair from the kitchen table.

"So Hon, what happened in school today?"

"Ah nuthin," came his usual reply.

After this answer, which I guess was supposed to pacify me, Paul trudged into the dining room to assemble his *GI Joe* toys. Moments later he returned and stood in the doorway. I noticed a brooding expression in his grey-blue eyes.

"What's on your mind?"

"Nuthin'."

Heading back to his chair he plunked himself down again. "Mom…"

"Yes…"

"Do you remember the time in Burlington when the doctor called to tell you that you were very sick?"

Foreboding caught in my throat. I lay down my paring knife. "What about it?"

"Well… I saw you put your head down and cry."

Oh no, I thought. I had always tried to save my crying jags for those times when the boys were out of the house.

"Go on." I prodded.

The next thing revealed by my solemn little boy distressed me even more. He went on in his no-nonsense way.

"Well, then I heard you say, 'I'm going to die, I'm going to die.'"

I gasped. "Paul, how could you have known that? I clearly remember that you were playing at Angela's house that morning!"

Paul played with the salt and peppershakers, making each one spin on its side. "I came home to find a toy… and that's when I heard you." He flicked each bottle harder.

"Oh, Paul," I sighed. My hand passed over the revolving missiles as though it would stop the spinning of our hearts too. "You were never meant to hear that. I thought I was all alone when I broke down like that."

"It's okay, Mom," he shrugged. "I know now that you're not going to die."

Abruptly, he left the kitchen signalling the end of our conversation. He returned to his war game while I numbly resumed scraping carrots. My mind peeled away layers of silent grief.

So that's why our youngest son had stuck so close to me during the past few years. We had wondered what triggered his withdrawn behaviour. Was it his grandpa Morgan's sudden death before we moved west? Was it the discovery of my disease? Or was it merely an expression of his "lone wolf" temperament? Whatever the cause we had not been able to persuade Paul to leave the house to play with friends after school as he had done before.

Now he had exposed his strategy of protection.

I turned to watch Paul through the doorway, his narrow frame sprawled on the carpet. Noisily he manoeuvred his plastic men dressed in army fatigues, around table legs and chairs.

"Hih, hih, hih!" His imaginary machine guns coughed relentlessly, as he defended his *GI Joe* troops from Enemy Cobra attacks. His bifocal glasses gradually crept closer to the ledge of his upturned nose until they rested on his pudgy cheeks.

I wanted to rush over and hug him to myself. But any sign of affection uninitiated by Paul would not be cool. That poor little boy, I groaned. He should never have had to carry such an oppressive burden. But he had finally exposed his secret because something had reassured him I was getting well.

Later that evening he snuggled next to me as our family shared popcorn and a funny show. A few weeks later Paul asked me if he could sleep over at a school friend's house.

The emotional healing had begun.

~

chapter 8
Mud of disillusionment, banner of glory, rhythms of life

When Ron suggested I take a break and fly to Ontario to see my family, my mentor-friend, Marge, asked if I would be open to a healing service at our home church. She said the pastors and deacons would be happy to lay hands on me for healing. Ron and I decided this would be worthwhile.

Ken and Cathy were present to witness and take part in stretching forth their hands with other brothers and sisters in Christ, asking God if He would restore my shrunken kidneys. An outrageous thing to ask of our Creator but surely He was still in the business of healing broken bodies.

After the service I pointed out the unsightly bulges on my dialysis arm to Cathy.

"Maybe God will heal these scars too," I sighed, rolling my sleeve back down. Though I was learning to accept my arm and even laugh about it with my sons, I did long for a smooth arm again.

Cathy touched my arm. "This is your badge of courage, Liz. Do not try to hide it."

Back home in my prairie dialysis unit I declared without reservation that a healing was in progress. "Soon I won't be needing dialysis anymore." I was certain God would want to showcase His power by healing a trusting child so that others would put their faith in Him.

Nurses and patients alternated between hoping for me, humouring me, and warning me not to get caught up in false hope.

When the months yielded no results I hit bottom. So what had been the point of this exercise in trust? I felt like a fool for telling people and for trusting God. What good could possibly come from His failure to come through?

Was I wrong to conclude God had failed? Had I misunderstood His promises in scripture that we would have whatever we asked for by faith in His Name?

No answers jumped out at me. Meanwhile I needed to settle down to the hard facts. I would be doing this tri-weekly routine for another five years and my family would be sharing the burden with me. No miracles in sight. No miracles to convince others that God is active in our world.

The wheels on my wagon of trust were stuck in the mud of disillusionment. I concluded it was up to God to decide how He would respond to my confusion. And it was up to me to pay attention. Meanwhile, I would carry on with this life as it was.

~

On one particular morning after bussing to Regina Hospital and needling my arm, I resumed my practice of reading a few verses in my Bible and asking God to show me what He wanted me to know.

Waiting for insight, I studied several of my fellow patients: Joe, always joking despite the loss of a leg, Barb, a young diabetic mother losing her morale, Stan a forty-something, handsome man of quiet faith grown gaunt from years of dialysis — all of them sitting in their *La-Z-Boy* chairs, with blood zipping through their lines to an artificial filter then returning cleaner blood to their bodies. I despaired for all of them. What kind of way was this to live? Why was I among them? Dear God, why?

As I prayed, a cloth banner came to mind: the banner I had noticed a few years earlier back in Toronto while leaving St. Michael's Hospital in a similar blur of disbelief. The embroidered words came back to me: *Bloom Where You Are Planted.*

Not exactly the answer I wanted or expected. Yet it gripped me.

Maybe... God had *planted* me in this dialysis ward and other wards to come. Maybe... it was no mistake that I was here. Could this setting be part of God's bigger plan?

Okay then, please show me how to bloom in this place, I pleaded.

A passage in Isaiah 61: 2-3 helped me to understand what blooming means. I read about the coming Jesus and His plan for us: "to give them beauty for ashes, the oil of joy for mourning, the garment of praise for the spirit of heaviness; that they may be called trees of righteousness, the planting of the Lord, that He may be glorified."

So blooming is about glorifying Him in whatever place I am planted!

Day by day, God showed me that to bloom or glorify Him meant to live by faith in this place.

If a person who belongs to Jesus lets His light shine in her, then she is blooming for His glory. Not always waiting for miracles, but living out the miracle of God's spiritual health; the health of trusting dependence upon Him.

My eyes fell back on Stan; he seemed to be blooming in this place. His eyes, hollowed by pain, held a divine kind of care for fellow patients and staff. Not stalled in self-pity, he would stop at each chair to pass on an encouraging word before starting his own dialysis regime, one he had lived for decades.

I too would learn how to take up the challenge of accepting these dreary places of suffering — where inmates mark time — as my divine calling. With the help of God's Spirit I would learn my new vocation. He would give me His beauty for ashes, His oil of joy for mourning, His garment of praise for the spirit of heaviness, to share with others.

~

I recalled someone else who knew a thing or two about illness and learning to trust in God. During our last year in Ontario before my kidney diagnosis I expressed great anxiety about my mysterious symptoms to my Southern Baptist neighbour, Mary.

A 49-year-old wife and mother to six young adults, Mary was fighting her third round with bowel cancer. She told me that well-meaning people were urging her to go to this and that healing service; to claim her healing, even to demand it of God as her right.

"But," she explained in her soft Georgian drawl, " I don't have to do that, I don't have to go running and begging like a frantic chicken." Her face glowed. "I just climb up onto the Lord's lap and I say, 'Daddy, I'm hurting.'" Then I tell Him how I wish that He would fix this sick old body so I don't have to leave yet."

Mary's blue eyes clouded up as they lingered on the family photo near her. "Still I know that His plans may be different from mine… and better!"

Angry tears escaped my eyes. It didn't seem fair that this loving person should suffer so much. Earlier that day I had watched Mary and her husband playing badminton with the small church group they had planted in our neighbourhood. These two sweethearts of thirty years exchanged glances filled with tenderness and laughter, each knowing the time could be short.

Squeezing my hand she smiled. "I'm just going to keep sitting in His lap. It's safe here, no matter what happens."

Within the year Mary died. She had gone to be in Jesus' presence forever.

From the vantage point of my dialysis chair I looked back and considered the lessons learned from her life. Did Mary's "Daddy" let her down? She would answer no. Her dying did not cancel out the wisdom of her choice to trust God. Nor did it diminish her influence on those she left behind.

~

Ron's contract with the troubled store he was hired to bring out of the red had been successfully completed. Applying his outstanding skills in management and inventory control, he had turned a failing business into a prosperous enterprise for its owner. Time to search for new conquests. And time to move past Moose Jaw, a place that taught us more than we could fathom then.

Possibilities for buying our own franchise opened up in Manitoba but a virus at the Health Sciences renal unit slammed that door shut. In early spring of 1984 another door opened in Taber, Alberta. It felt like someone had pulled back the curtains and opened the windows to let in the sunshine and invite the breezes to blow through.

Ron finally got the hardware store he had dreamed and worked toward since he was a lad of fifteen working for Spencer's Hardware in Oakville, Ontario. Soon our family of four became part of the enterprise, dusting and stocking shelves, pricing stock as it arrived, waiting on customers and enjoying the quaintness of another small town.

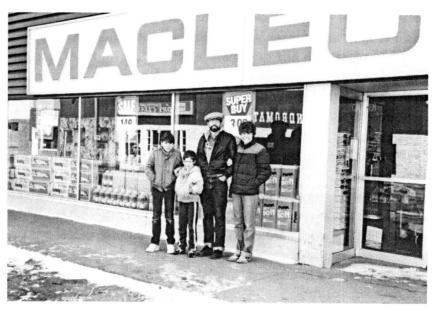

We four work at our new franchise, Taber 1984

Since my Lethbridge dialysis unit was only forty-five minutes away, Ron and I wondered if I had developed the endurance to drive myself there and back. After a few test runs we were thrilled to see how far I had come. These solitary trips allowed me a greater measure of autonomy. Still nervous about inserting my own needles I found the scenes of grain elevators and farmers' fields along the highway a refreshing distraction. After my nurses helped me get hooked up to my lifeline I brought out my notepad and Bible to write stories about these scenes and ponder the ways God was helping my life to move forward.

~

When one of my nurses noticed my journaling habits, she suggested I find a writers' group in Taber to see if I had a talent. Seemed like a fun idea to explore. But what if they thought I had nothing worth reading? I read a few poems to them and hoped I could accept their verdict without getting too down on myself. Some in the group encouraged me to sign up for writing courses taught at night by Hazel West, a dynamic high school teacher. I thought, *why not explore this avenue!* Through this course I made some new friends. One of them became irate on my behalf when she noted that the teacher had picked apart my writing more than that of other classmates.

So, it had not been my imagination! Maybe Mrs. West didn't like my style, or me. Ron countered that maybe she expected more from me than the others. A phone call from my instructor cleared up the matter. I could hardly believe what she was proposing.

"How would you like to join a select group of serious writers who assist one another in getting their work published?"

This was like a little bit of heaven. Someone saw possibilities for me. Echoes of the past: my mom had predicted I would become a teacher and then a writer. More recently, Jacquie, my social worker, had urged me to write a book. Could these be road signs for me to follow?

Hazel was tireless in her encouragement and demand for excellence; our group gave practical support to one another. One night I read them a short inspirational piece called, *Another Chance with Mom*, about my mother's brush with death a few years earlier. They agreed it would be a good fit for a Catholic family magazine in North Battleford. So I learned the protocol for submitting an article and sent it off. That was an exciting moment for me as I wondered where it might take me.

~

My anticipation was muted by news from home. Dad called from Oakville, his voice low and gentle. My mom's brave battle with liver disease and rheumatoid arthritis was over. We had received a number of calls over the years to say that Mom was near death, but this time it was final. She was gone. I paced and wept. I needed to do something, go somewhere…

I aimed the car toward my fellow writing friend's farm. Chris had urged me to come visit her on this damp March morning. She met me at the door with a pair of galoshes. I pulled them on and followed her to an A-frame barn in the field. The muddy snow squished and slid beneath my feet. This seemed a strange way to give me comfort but my friend made no explanation. When we arrived, she invited me to have a look in the straw. There lay a ewe, nursing her newborn lambs. We stood in silence watching this miracle of birth that never fails to move the human spirit.

The rhythms of life carry on. Life and death and life, again. We trudged back the way we came and sipped steaming tea in my friend's kitchen.

~

Every so often on Sundays after church we enjoyed taking our boys out for a buffet lunch in Lethbridge. Mark, age twelve, preferred we sit in a corner near a potted palm where he would not be noticed in case he had food stuck in his teeth. At his age looking cool mattered.

During our meal, he began rocking his chair back and forth. "Mark, you may rock back too far and tip over," his dad warned. Mark assured us he was being careful. He continued to tilt his chair. Suddenly all we saw of him were his feet pointing straight up. Our cool son and his chair became part of the palm tree.

Poor Mark. We waited to see what he would do. From the floor there came a rumble of laughter. Then we heard diners around us laughing. And when Mark came up, they clapped. Nice one, Mark. Now everyone is watching you.

Paul, age eight, could not resist mocking his big brother. He returned to the buffet and came back with a sprig of lettuce hanging from his mouth — to simulate Mark eating palm leaves for his brunch. We had more laughs at Mark's expense. He should have listened to his father.

~

It had been three months since Mom had passed away. I was trying to work the cranky till at our store when Ron stopped, leaned over and handed me an envelope. "Open it now, Hon."

The return address: *Our Family* magazine. Ripping the envelope apart, I found a brief letter thanking me for my submission. Oh yes, I had been warned about these terse messages from the editor to let us down easy. Reading the next line I yelped and wept. Never mind what the poor customer thought of my fitful performance. Ron reached over to read it too. "We would like to publish your piece in our summer issue… "

Laughing with me, Ron held me close, and kissed my hair, "I knew you had it in you — the gift to move people with your writing."

I thought, how appropriate that my first published story would be about my recently deceased mother who had planted within me the seeds of possibility.

I could hear my mother saying it again to me. "Elizabeth, one day you will become a writer."

~

chapter 9
writing flurry, sober responsibility, self-sacrificing husband

My dialysis routine began to take on a life of its own, a place reserved for my writing hours. Ron bought me a typewriter that accompanied me three times a week to dialysis in Lethbridge. While other patients dozed in their chairs for their three- to four-hour runs I pecked away at the keys, eager to see what words and ideas would transfer from my mind to paper.

At regular intervals a dialysis technician came to our unit to repair our dialysis machines. As he worked on the machine near me, he began a dialogue that would lead to some surprising outcomes.

"Whenever I come here I notice that you are writing or typing. What do you write about?"

I told him that I journal about my family and what it's like to be on dialysis — always dependent on the medical system for the rest of my life.

"I have a friend who publishes and edits a professional renal magazine in Toronto, called *Renal Family*," he informed me. "It's written by medical people but I think he should let patients give their input."

I had never seen or heard of the magazine until he found a copy on a rack for me to peruse.

Pointing his wrench at me, he said, "Why don't you submit something you've written and see what he thinks. All he can do is turn it down or consider it."

When I relayed the conversation to Ron he was all for the idea. What a gift that I could count on my love to cheer me on wherever he saw an opportunity for growth.

A few weeks later the phone rang in the dialysis unit. A nurse answered it and extended the cord to reach me. "It's for you. Someone called Lorne."

"Hello?"

"Hello, this is Lorne Cooper of *Renal Family* magazine. I received your piece and read it."

"Yes… " I waited to hear his verdict while my heart did somersaults. He wouldn't be calling if he didn't have an interest, I thought. The story had been about the scenes that calm my spirit as I travel along the highway leading to my dialysis unit.

"I didn't really care for the story."

"Oh," My spirit drooped. *Then why was he calling?*

"However, I would like to see what else you might have to write about the dialysis life itself, the challenges and so on. Would you write me a 1200-word essay for the next issue?"

I blubbered. I dithered. "I have to think about it."

"Yes, or no."

Oh what a coward! The publisher of a magazine is asking for a commitment and I'm dumbstruck.

"Uhhh… yes!" I spit it out again before I could back out, "Yes!"

"Good. I'd like to see it in a month."

~

What happy confusion! One month to produce a piece and send it off. I had a lot of work to do. What to write about next? He wanted any topic relating to the difficulties of living with renal failure and the dialysis routine. My recent experiences in trying to travel to Toronto and Florida and arrange dialysis appointments along the way provided plenty of dilemmas. Ron assisted me in mapping out the article.

When the quarterly magazine arrived (along with a cheque) and several complimentary copies I passed them around to my cheering squad of nurses and fellow patients at dialysis. We thumbed our way to the article titled, *The Traveller's Dilemma: A Patient's Perspective* by Liz Morgan. They were generous in their congratulations.

Ron and I were absolutely delighted with how God was opening windows right and left for us. What happened to me happened to my family as well. And now we prayed that our experiences would bless others who were going through similar hard times.

~

The crowning touch came when Mr. Cooper called again with another proposal. He said that my article covered the type of material he thought added value to his magazine for renal professionals and wondered if I would like to write under the title of *From A Patient's Perspective*.

When I wasn't clear on what he was suggesting he clarified. "I would like you to write for every quarterly."

He was offering me my own column! This time he gave me time to talk it over with Ron since it would require a long-term commitment.

Ron encouraged me to accept the column as another part of God's placement for me. Although I had often regretted missing most dialysis parties because I did not have the emotional energy for them, my fellow patients' trials were an ever-present sorrow for me. Ron pointed out that writing about the challenges of the dialysis life was a useful way to serve my fellow patients — by writing on behalf of all of us. Maybe in this way greater understanding of our dilemmas would deliver better care for all of us.

I accepted the offer with joy and sober responsibility. God and I and my Ron, we could do this, one article at a time. This offer presented me with another way to bloom in the place God had planted me.

~

Things had not gone in our favour regarding our first franchise, so Ron cut his losses and set his sights on a hardware franchise with a different company in a different town. The town of Wetaskiwin, Alberta, fifty minutes south of Edmonton, offered inviting possibilities.

But first Ron wanted to ensure that dialysis was provided in that town, to eliminate the travel factor. An accident enroute to dialysis in Lethbridge had motivated this decision. One winter at dawn, I had spun out of control on black ice. My van crossed the median and plowed into a ditch after a light standard smashed into my passenger side, popping out the back windows. No injury to me, but the van sustained considerable damage.

Our fact-finding mission took us to the dialysis chiefs at University of Alberta Hospital in Edmonton. A lot rode on this enquiry. If our mission proved unsuccessful, Ron committed himself to search for another town and another enterprise. As I write this account I give thanks that God gave me such a self-sacrificing husband to watch over me.

The shortest version of the story is that due to the high density of renal patients in the surrounding area, a Wetaskiwin unit was promised to us in order to service many patients like me. We were assured that we could base our move on the administration's word.

In good faith we moved to Wetaskiwin in January of '86. For several months I travelled tri-weekly to dialysis in Edmonton, understanding this arrangement was temporary. However, due to budget cutbacks the Wetaskiwin project was withdrawn.

Deeply disappointed, we decided not to give up. For several weeks I "camped" on the office doorstep of the key renal doctor who could pull strings. With gentle but persistent pleas I urged him to find a way to come through. After several reasonable meetings he and his staff found a way to keep their promise.

~

It mattered not to me that a small, unused laundry room in the basement of the aging Wetaskiwin Hospital — formerly a nursing residence — became my dialysis home. We received this humble setting as a generous gift. No more long drives to dialysis.

In addition, so many area patients got transplants that I usually had the two-machine unit to myself. I had the luxury of my very own dialysis nurse, Dianne, who became my advocate and dear friend, partnering with me in my writing endeavours as well as my health care. She often asked me to read aloud what I had written for the next *Renal Family* quarterly. Together we discussed changes or additional perspectives for future issues. This friend made my years on dialysis a place of friendship and laughter.

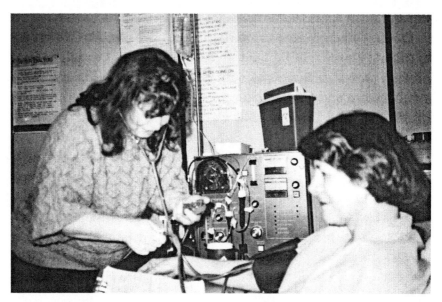

Dialysing with my nurse Dianne in a former laundry room, Wetaskiwin 1986

While fellow patients quickly qualified for transplants, my five-year wait for a kidney extended to many more years than predicted. Many people helped me to manage this lifestyle with acceptance.

A woman from our church, Leslie, who had heard about my health challenges, came to pay me several visits. Eventually she came every Wednesday for years and we became very good friends. I could always count on Leslie to offer a shoulder, practical insight, side-splitting laughter and prayers.

Another new friend Nettie, who was a hospital library technician, dropped by nearly every dialysis day to chat a while. Though other staff hurried to their workstations, Nettie took time to enquire about my treatment and wellbeing. She arranged for me to give in-service seminars about dialysis from a patient's perspective to hospital staff. As well, nursing instructors from Lacombe and

Camrose schools came with their students to observe my dialysis regime. These visits turned into dual learning sessions, one in the dialysis room and one in a nearby classroom. On a dialysis day I explained the dialysis routine while I inserted my own needles and they observed the cleansing process. Some students fainted the first time. Remembering my own initial reactions, I could certainly identify with them.

The following day I met with them in class to explain the technical side of kidney failure, using charts and chalkboard. To lighten these sessions ten-year-old Paul drew a series of cartoon flashcards depicting the side effects of kidney failure. A caricature of his mom with head in toilet titled, *Nausea*, is just one example that provided hilarity. These were mutually stimulating sessions with many questions about the personal and spiritual side of coping with kidney failure and chronic illness. My articles written for *Renal Family* became part of their renal education. These young women and men gave me great encouragement as they expressed gratitude for the help they received through our contacts.

Dianne and I always looked forward to bi-annual visits from my academic aunts from Calgary. Betty and Dorothy came every so often bearing gifts of muffins, cookies, beet borscht, and stories of their overseas travels to share during my dialysis run. Their no-nonsense presence always gave us encouragement for our own journeys. They expressed pride in Ron and me for how we got on with life, and assured us of their prayers.

Most of all my husband and sons provided me with constant love and support and a lot of laughter, too. I enjoyed documenting some of our funnier moments.

~

I was in our main bathroom when I heard a tap on the door. "M-o-m, how long are you going to be?"

"Use the other bathroom," I called.

"I don't need to get in. I'm just waiting to show you something I got at the mall."

"Well, hold on Mark."

"Okay," he sighed. But he didn't leave the door. I heard him whispering to someone and laughing.

I finally opened the door and saw his buddy, Corey, standing next to Mark.

The two strapping fifteen-year-old boys grinned nervously.

"So, Mom, what do you think?"

"About what?" I studied Mark up and down, and then up again. Yikes! What I saw was one very raw, inflamed ear. With an earring in it!

Now mother take it easy, I counseled myself. *Don't react. It's just an earring.*

"Do you think Dad will mind?" Mark asked.

Oh ya, he will mind! I thought to myself — but made no comment.

"Do you think it looks good on me?"

"Sure Mark," I tried not to smirk. "It looks fine." Flaming red but fine.

Just then his adolescent brother, Paul, rounded the corner, assessed the situation and quipped, "Hey Mark, it *does* look good! I always wanted a sister!"

We all broke up, including Mark, who tried to take a swipe at Paul — but was laughing too hard to snag him.

~

chapter 10
Wearing out, jazzing up, hearing Jesus

By the twelfth year of dialysis I began to show the wear and tear of this demanding medical intervention. Toxins in my blood were not clearing efficiently, bones in my feet and ribcage were breaking spontaneously — the latter during a mammogram — and my morale took a detour into clinical depression and daily panic attacks that lasted for ten suffocating months.

Often while we were driving to Edmonton for doctors' appointments in the dead of winter, I would roll the window down to gulp in fresh air. I could not bear to be closed in — not in the van, bathroom or other small spaces.

In addition, a new hospital had been built in our town and my dialysis nurse and friend, Dianne, found another job in her rural town, while I moved into the new dialysis unit with three new nurses to serve about ten additional patients. I missed the familiarity of my laundry room setting and my own nurse.

~

Throughout these harder times, Ron and I continued our weekly restaurant dates. But we needed a new kind of distraction. One evening he shared an idea he had been pondering.

"Hon, I've always had an interest in jazz," Ron began. "I've been thinking that we could drive into Edmonton to take in a jazz event. Do you want to give it a try?"

Oh yes, I was game for a new diversion. Ron had bought me some lovely new outfits for fine dining and I loved dressing up and looking my best.

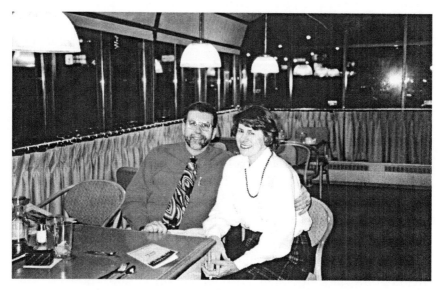

Dressing up and dining out 1995

Our first exposure to JazzFest had us hooked. We decided to find smaller venues in cozy bistros where we could sit near the front for the best sound and view. Since we sat right near the band and singers, they often joined us during their breaks. We added a new set of friends to our life, people who gave hugs freely. At first we held back from their affectionate gestures but after a while we became huggers too, appreciating their sincerity and the chance to affirm one another.

To enhance our enjoyment of these outings, Ron rented a tiny bachelor apartment in an Edmonton high-rise where we could retreat for a whole weekend of jazz events. How I enjoyed sitting close to Ron who was always attentive, holding my hand or whispering sweet appreciation into my ear, while we watched each performance. Sometimes, Ron would ask one of our friends to dedicate a song to me. Tears clouded our eyes when Kennedy Jenson sang, *First Time Ever I Saw Your Face*, for us. Debbie Boodram, Dianne

Donovan, Sue Moss and Anna Beaumont were other special friends who dedicated many songs for us.

These outings led to expanding friendships that were later proven as my health continued to decline. During one of my hospitalizations for a serious kidney infection, four women who had created their own group, *Wine Women and Song*, noted that Ron had come alone to hear them sing. They were very concerned and the morning after their inaugural gig they surprised me with a hospital visit, bringing flowers and songs. Ron and I felt honoured by their genuine expressions of care.

~

When my nighttime disturbances with restless leg syndrome and panic attacks continually kept Ron awake, we decided I would move across the hall into our spare office/bedroom. If my husband were to help me through all the daytime challenges of my failing health and running his business he needed to get his rest. Often our sheltie, Skimmer, crawled under my bed, especially when she sensed I was very ill.

It was on one such night when I felt overwhelmed by my long sojourn of panic and weakness that I sat up in my office bed and began screaming. Ron could not hear me and Mark had already left home for college in Victoria but Paul was still at home and his bedroom was directly below the spare room. I heard his long legs bounding up the stairway.

"Mom? Are you all right?"

"Yes… no… I am frightened."

My son sat in the chair at the foot of my bed and waited for me to talk, or not. That was his way.

"I'm afraid of dying in my sleep." I explained. 'These panic attacks cause me to feel like I will suffocate."

Paul said nothing as I talked. During the hour or so I eventually ran out of words and fell silent and then asleep.

After a few times of this night encounter with my son, I grew used to the rhythm; he would sit quietly and wait, then slip out when I had exhausted myself. One night when I had nothing more to say and began to doze, I heard Paul's bones creak as he stood up to leave.

At that moment, our routine – me talking, my son listening — struck me as very funny.

"Hey, Paul," I called out.

He stopped.

"One of these days you will make a lot of money doing this… listening to people."

We grinned. You never knew what could come from hard times, a career choice perhaps.

~

When Ron suggested the source of my panic could be related to menopause, I sought the advice of a gynaecologist who put me on a hormone patch and referred me to a female psychologist. I was agreeable to this referral. I wanted to end the terror I was experiencing and putting all of us through.

At first the psychologist wanted to hypnotize me. I asked her not do that since I did not want to give the power of my mind over to anyone but God. She heeded my request and won me over to the idea of an imagination session where I could write the scene.

Dr. Pam invited me to lie down on a couch while she closed the blinds and turned off the lights. After a few sessions I had already agreed to let her close her office door — a big deal for me as my sweat glands heated up. I wanted to flee her office, run outside and breathe. Instead I lay still while she played a CD of soothing pipe music. As usual I asked God to protect my mind from anything that was not from Him. She instructed me that whatever I saw or heard was for me alone and not to tell her during this exercise.

"I want you to close your eyes and imagine yourself in a place that makes you feel safe and peaceful."

My mind travelled to a seashore in Victoria along Dallas Road. I sat on a log listening to the water lapping against the rocks.

She spoke in quiet tones helping me to create the scene of restfulness.

"You are alone with your peaceful thoughts when you see someone approaching you."

I stiffened.

"Oh no, you are not afraid at all. Even though this person is still too far off to recognize, it is a friend you will be happy to see."

I let my muscles sink back into the couch. I was sure it was my sweetheart, Ron.

"Now they are getting closer and you finally see who it is."

I was caught by the unexpected. It was not Ron at all. It was Jesus! Jesus of the cross and of my life!

"This person is saying something to you. It is something you are glad to hear."

I waited to hear what He would say. "I will never leave you nor forsake you."

That simple promise and nothing more. Oh, these words were so lovely to hear. They were the sound of water washing over a rocky place.

The psychologist remained quiet for so long I wondered if she had slipped out of the room.

Had I wept? I don't remember. I only knew that Jesus would never leave me and had never left me. I knew He was healing this panic and that soon I would no longer be requiring this good doctor's services.

She finally crept into the sacred silence, gradually opening the blinds and asking me to open my eyes again. "I know I told you not to tell me but I wonder if you would like to reveal who it was you saw… The reason I ask is because the most wonderful smile flowed over your face."

I told her it was Jesus — my place of safety.

Within the month my panic attacks dissipated like the mists that hang low in our Edmonton river valley and then lift as the sunshine burns through.

~

chapter 11
Excruciating time, angelic blessings, long-suffering son

I had still to deal with the fact that my dialysis no longer functioned well for me. Short walks around our little crescent left me winded. I was turning sallow, losing weight and so very weary. My friends could no longer hide the look of dread they felt for me. A nurse in my dialysis unit had whispered too loudly to another nurse, "I don't think she will make it".

My Edmonton specialist recommended I turn to my family tree once more and search for a kidney transplant donor. He pointed out that drug therapies had vastly improved, making it more feasible that my system might accept a far-from-ideal match. He underlined the fact that a related living donor was my best chance for survival.

Paul had moved to Edmonton in order to attend Bible College for a year. When he learned that my doctor advised I approach my siblings again, he said he wanted to be tested first. Everything in this mother's heart objected. I could not let my son give up one of his organs for me. He was only nineteen. It was my job to watch out for him, not the other way around! But it seemed to be a task Paul had chosen to take on.

Paul informed me he would help and that was the end of the matter. How relieved I felt when preliminary tests revealed our blood type was not a match.

Among my siblings, those with good health — Susan and Dave — came forward for testing. Ron and I were touched by these generous offers from family and even from friends. In case no family members matched, we had several friends who waited to be tested: Leslie and her daughter Alyson, plus two members of Ron's staff.

To relieve the tension of this waiting period we decided to head to Victoria for a short winter break.

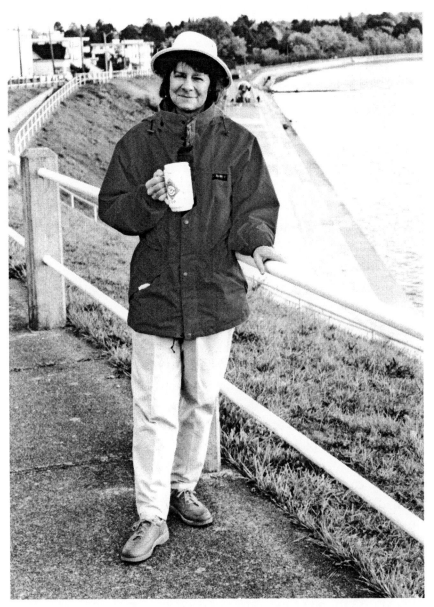

Time out on Dallas Road coast while waiting for donor match, Victoria 1996

Walks along Dallas Road coast would do us good. While dialysing in the Hillside clinic there, I noted the various visitors coming and going, and pondered who in my family would turn out to be the closest match. My stomach churned at the thought of a transplant with all its risks. But I knew I could not carry on much longer on dialysis.

Another visitor walked into the clinic, a dark-haired young man wearing a beret. Watching his confident stride I gasped when he stopped in front of my chair.

"Hi Mom," he grinned kissing my cheek and hugging me lightly, mindful of all the bloodlines in my left arm tethering me to the filtering machine.

"Mark! I thought you were in film class." My twenty-three-year-old son had moved to Victoria to attend chef school but switched to film instead.

"Ya, I took some time off — I wanted to see you since this will be one of your last dialysis treatments. Pretty soon you won't have to do this anymore."

I knew it made Mark feel physically ill to see me on this machine all these years. As we talked I confessed I was feeling pretty intimidated by the next step.

With tears clouding his eyes, my son told me he knew I could get through a transplant just the way I got through thirteen years of dialysis. "Mom, it is because I have watched you surviving all this stuff that I know I can handle anything in life, too."

Now it was my turn to tear up. Mark's words bolstered my morale. If my son could picture both of us enduring anything, then these medical trials were building fibre in all of us.

At the end of my last dialysis run in Victoria I received the news we had anticipated. My older brother, Dave, was found to be the only viable match. This was really going to happen. We flew home the next day to begin the lengthy tedious workup process for this long-awaited kidney transplant.

My specialist cautioned us that the match was not great because of my rare antibodies so the risk of rejection was high. Dave did not care if his kidney donation failed — he wanted at least to try. When the week for surgery approached we met my brother at Edmonton International airport. "You look good, Sis," he said kindly, hiding his distress at my depleted condition.

Years later I learned of a moving conversation that had taken place as Dave sat outside the University Hospital with a high school buddy, Hilford who had flown out from BC to support Dave. My brother had grieved over how gaunt and worn I looked. He feared I would die. So did others.

It must have been an excruciating time for my Ron, Mark and Paul, my dad, our family tree and all others who cared for us. Everyone put on a brave front and earnestly sought God's intervention. Even Dave's ex-girlfriend called from England where she holidayed with her mom whom I had never met. This mother and daughter had knelt at their hotel bed asking God to guard brother and sister in surgery and afterwards.

~

The evening before surgery remains vague for me except for one clear image. Several came to pray with me, and in the midst of this Dave appeared in the doorway. I had not expected to see him before surgery.

Looking solemn, he handed me a mug with the Footprint story printed on it. A man had dreamed that often in his life there were two sets of footprints in the sand, but during the lowest points there was only one set. When he asked the Lord about His promise to walk with him all the way, the Lord explained. "My precious, precious child. I love you and would never leave you. During your times of trial and suffering when you see only one set of footprints, it was then that I carried you." God was using Dave to carry me.

Then my brother also handed me a cloth-covered book. "For your journaling," he said, "I thought you might want to write about this time some day."

How incredibly thoughtful. Wasn't it enough that he had flown across the country to submit himself to surgery and the sacrifice of a vital organ! He kissed me goodbye and returned to his ward.

When the buzz of night preps died away I opened the blank journal. Inside the cover my third oldest brother had scribbled these words: "To my dear sister Liz, from Dave with love. God be with you. April 30, 1996."

I was moved. My brother was not demonstrative with his affection and faith. He was practical but I sensed the tender emotion behind the gifts.

~

DAYS ONE AND TWO
May 1, 1996.

When morning broke I thought about what was about to transpire. My body was failing me and I wondered if I would make it, and if I wanted to make it.

I feared more deadly weariness, the suffering after surgery, the chance of developing a moon face and facial hair growth from the powerful anti-rejection drugs. I feared kidney rejection and return to dialysis for the rest of my days.

Then I turned my thoughts to my brother and what he was experiencing this day. I thought about him in clinical terms because if I let myself slide down the emotional route, I would be a mess. He would proceed to surgery ahead of me to have one of his kidneys removed. The surgeon would cut through muscle and break a rib to get at it. Then the precious organ would be placed on ice until I was prepped to receive it in an adjoining room.

The original plan was for two teams of surgeons to perform our surgery — one team to remove one of Dave's kidney and another team to open my abdomen — so that the organ could be placed in me with the shortest time in transit. The longer an organ remains on ice the more quickly it begins to deteriorate.

But, the previous night, after Dave's visit, I had been informed that the second team was required for another transplant. I was given the option to back out and wait for another surgical date. After a quick consult, Ron and I decided we did not want to delay the procedure any further. We would trust God with the outcome.

~

As I was wheeled into the surgical room, I shivered. The place felt like an icebox. Gowned and gloved staff buzzed around me preparing the surgical supplies and talking in low tones amongst themselves. *Someone please talk to me! I am terrified.* Of course they could not hear my silent cries. Ron sat downstairs praying for Dave and me, and for our surgical team.

Lord, if it's okay with you... I'm so very weary... please will you let me go?

The answer that returned to my spirit came with sure conviction. *You will suffer much but you will live.* It was settled. This was God's will for me and my family.

Hands touched me. Draped me in green. Painted my pelvic area orange — not my best colour. Slapped my right arm to bring up veins, to insert IV's. A voice said to start counting backwards from ten. I knew this drill; I welcomed it. This sensation of drifting away before I could finish six... Then, sweet release.

"Mrs. Morgan, wake up, it's all over."

"Owww, it hurts... quick, a basin!"

~

A team of doctors went to find my husband. When Ron saw the grave posse approaching him his gut started to turn over. Why four doctors? Why not just one?

"Mr. Morgan, your wife is in the recovery room now."

Ron wanted them to get on with the facts. "What happened?"

"We don't know what went wrong. The new kidney started up as soon as we hooked your wife up to it. Right away it was producing urine, but by the time we finished sewing her up... the graft stopped working."

"So what does this mean?"

"We have to wait and see if it will start working again. Right now the graft has gone into shock."

~

We were in shock, too. Soul-wrenching shock.

Why had this new kidney stopped working? We were told possibly because of the need for high doses of powerful anti-rejection drugs to prevent my immune system from rejecting a foreign organ. Doses can be too high or not enough. Fine-tuning is required. We considered that the graft might have been on ice too long during the transition from Dave's body to mine.

Day one passed, then day two, while we waited for the kidney to produce urine. I was instructed to go into the washroom every few hours to try to pee. Maybe the graft would start up. But nothing happened. Making and passing urine was something my body had not been able to do for nearly thirteen years. Failed kidneys do not produce urine and dialysis does not produce urine; the treatment only removes the toxins that were once removed by a functioning kidney.

~

Early mornings found Paul sitting at my bedside with an oversized Bible in his lap as he studied for his Bible School classes. When he left mid-morning, his father arrived for the next shift with coffee mug in one hand and the *Globe and Mail* in the other. As much as my love hated the hospital environment, he stayed by my side in one way or another. Whether Ron was working at his store or at home taking care of duties, or having his daily quiet time with the Lord, his motivation was always to see to my needs and pray through until they were met.

People round the globe — in Zambia, England, North Carolina, Oakville, Edmonton, Vancouver, and Australia — were enlisted by family and friends to also pray through on behalf of Ron and me, our sons, my brother, and our caregivers.

~

DAY THREE

Dave arrived, gripping his side where a rib had been broken to remove one of his healthy kidneys for my sake.

"How are you doing, Sis?" He had already heard how our kidney was doing. "I would have come sooner but I've been in a fair bit of pain."

I could see that. He sat crouched over, wincing between weak smiles. Though a tough, gruff guy, used to the rigors of deep sea diving as his trade, this pain was brutal even for him. Taking my hand my brother made an unusual proposition in all seriousness.

"I've been thinking about what to do if your kidney doesn't recover… "

What he suggested still amazes me.

"I would like to ask the surgeons if he they would take a part of my other kidney and transplant it into you."

I smiled at his offer. He protested that he was serious, that the technology to transplant a fraction of an organ might have already been developed. My brother, so gifted with a brilliant technical inventors' mind, had already designed impossible equipment for pouring concrete under water and using the technology in his contracts with Shell Oil. Ever since his teens he had been designing and stitching together his own diving suits.

The very fact that my brother-donor was offering to go through it again, to give me quality life — well, it left me speechless. After he hobbled back to his ward I shook my head in wonder. Wow, that visit was sweet no matter what happened next.

Later on day three, I had to be hooked back up to dialysis. Ron's spirits must have slumped when he saw me on the machine again. I told him the doctor hoped it would be a temporary measure until the kidney restarted itself.

~

DAYS FOUR AND FIVE

Paul wheeled me to the dialysis ward and to various tests to see what the kidney was doing. Each test revealed it was still in shock.

While I was being dialysed I felt so depressed I heard myself give shocking advice to a daughter whose aging mother was having a tough time on dialysis. "Why don't you let her go off dialysis and die?" Waving a hand at our equipment I whispered, "This is no life for her!"

When I returned to my room I wept as I told Ron about my discouraging words to a person who needed to be cheered on. When my meal tray arrived I insisted I couldn't eat a thing. Ron pushed the tray toward me. With every mouth full of casserole I let my tears roll freely and my complaints multiply.

Ron began to chuckle.

I looked up. "What?" I retorted defensively. He was grinning like a fool. "What is so darn funny?"

"You are, Hon. Look at you." Ron pointed at me scraping up the last morsel from my plate. "While you've been crying about how bad the drugs make you feel and act, I've watched you wolf down your entire meal. You practically licked your plate. You haven't eaten like that in months!"

I began to laugh, too. Silly me. Life does have its funny side, doesn't it?

~

DAY SIX

Mid-morning, Dave surprised me when he entered my hospital room looking handsome in his navy suit and a smile.

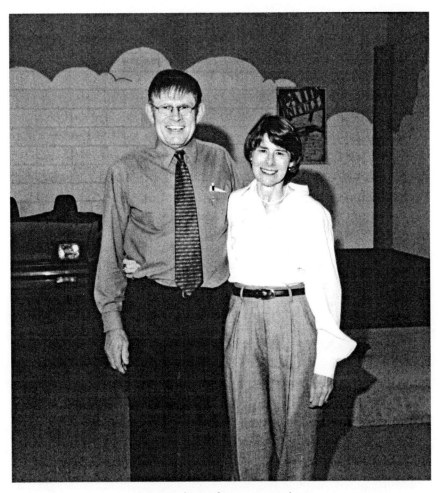

Dave and me after my transplant

It was time for his departure back to Oakville, Ontario where he ran his diving business. He held his side. It still hurt, but he was anxious to get back home. He kissed me goodbye and assured me of his prayers. As I watched my brother walk away with Ron I thought about the incomparable sacrifice he had made for me. *Lord, bless him as only You can.*

~

DAY SEVEN

As Paul stood by my stretcher parked outside another exam room, I wondered why he squinted up the corridor and then down the corridor. At that moment the hallway held no traffic. Only the two of us occupied it.

"Mom. Where is your transplant?" he asked in a low tone.

I patted my right side over my sheet. "Right here. Why?"

Then Paul lightly placed his hand on that area and bowed his head, his muscular frame towering over me. I heard no words but I sensed a holy conversation between my younger son and his God. My heart welled up in tears. The Lord was growing my son into a man of faith and prayer: a man of God.

~

DAY EIGHT: Part one

When Paul arrived for his morning vigil I said I couldn't face another lifetime on dialysis. Lying very still I wondered how my spirit would ever survive this. I wondered where my Lord had gone. Every day I had tried to pee but nothing came. Soon the doctors would have to remove my graft if nothing transpired.

Paul carried on with his studies, his grandpa Morgan's large-print Bible in his lap. After a time, he looked up and spoke to my grief.

"Mom… if you do have to stay on dialysis, God isn't trying to hurt you."

Only that one statement and then my son went back to his books. *God isn't trying to hurt you.* It was enough. Others had faith on my behalf when mine had run dry. What tenderness in my son's words of hope. What tenderness in the Father's care over us.

~

DAY EIGHT: Part two

Checking the clock on the wall — 9:30 am — I remembered it was time for my routine trip to the washroom. Might as well try.

142

Paul had to move his chair slightly so I could squeeze past his long legs to enter the washroom. Placing what they call a "hat" on the toilet seat, I sat down to wait for my miracle.

So many wonderful things were happening in the midst of this frightening time period that I would not want to miss. I thought of all the people who had come to my bedside to minister to my needs over recent days. So much love poured out to me from family and friends of every stripe. My family spread around the world ensured their churches and care groups prayed for all of us. Even strangers sent messages of encouragement.

Mark, who could not be present because he was completing film school in Victoria, sent me cards reminding me I can get through anything. To his reassuring words my son injected some humour that had me holding my side with laughter. One card with a grumpy woman on the cover said: *You should do what I do when I'm not feeling well... make life unbearable for everyone else!* In his note, he wrote: *Dear Mom, I'm sorry about the complications but I know that you will use them to your advantage. The fact that I know you're so strong, keeps me strong. I LOVE YOU!*

New friends from our jazz outings arrived. Anna brought a dozen red, long-stemmed roses, and with a fellow musician they serenaded me on a mandolin; Kennedy came to cheer me on; and Debbie read a psalm to me, knowing that I loved to read scripture.

One weary afternoon Ron was moved to tears when he entered my room and found another dear friend, Anita, and one of my dialysis nurses, Kathy, from Wetaskiwin General washing my hair. He called them angels of mercy, people who were helping him to watch over me. In one of many lovely cards Ron wrote: *Angels come in many forms. The Lord has sent legions of angels to care for you — seen and unseen. Liz this is the worst of times and the best of times!*

Many other angels came also bearing blessings: Dean and Kirsten who brought hope and knowledge — he as a medical researcher and she as a cherished friend from Ontario days. Kirsten had attended our youth group when Ron and I had taught the teen Bible class in Ontario. Loyal Leslie came despite her own suffering from a recent fall; Nettie humbly delivered hope with conviction through a dream where she saw me running — me who could hardly walk a block; and Hazel brought lotion and prayers to massage my dry limbs and spirit.

My musings ended when I felt an unusual sensation, one I had not experienced in nearly thirteen years. What was this?

Behold! A trickle of water.

Then, another trickle. And one more. I measured it — one teaspoon. It wasn't much, but it was something!

I washed my hands and cracked the door open, peering around it to meet my son's eyes.

"Did you hear that?" I whispered.

Paul nodded. "I am hoping it was what I thought it was," he said.

By now we were both grinning with joy. Just a few trickles but, boy, it was a good sound, the sound of music to our ears! The sound of hope.

I rang the call bell to inform my nurse.

~

DAY NINE

I passed another few drops. Ron wanted to be happy for me but he knew that more output would be needed, that my doctor would be looking for far more promising results. Ron knew how to keep me grounded so that I would be ready for disappointments while hoping for a brighter outcome.

My doctor confirmed Ron's practical observations. A small amount of output each day would not be enough to keep me off dialysis. It would take far more than that — cups and litres — but it was an encouraging sign.

~

DAY TEN

May 10, 1996.

A date to commemorate. Twenty-seven years earlier we had stood together; I trembling in my gown of too many ruffles [what had I been thinking!], my groom solemn in his tux. We gathered before the Lord, our pastor and our family and friends to declare our devotion and commitment to one another, to honour one another through sickness and health for as long as we lived.

Of course we had not known the trials we would face, but surely God knew and had been tutoring us every step of the way to stay close to Him. It was because of the Lord's faithful pursuit and guidance that we had made it this far in one piece. The tests seemed severe at times but wasn't God helping our love to mature? Yet sometimes I wasn't sure that we were okay.

Sometimes when Ron's expression seemed flat and distant, I fought back fears that he didn't care anymore. It had been a long, lonely road for him as well as for me. How many times had the doctor cautioned my husband that I might not make it? Many times, I suspected. How many times did he wonder whether this was the time he would be left alone with two young boys to raise?

When my love arrived he sat down on the chair beside me, his eyes wearing a weariness of soul.

I knew he dreaded these hospital visits — too many over the years — especially when there were few signs that I was getting well. When we were apart we yearned for one another. But in the hospital setting, Ron's morale froze; he wanted to get each visit over with and flee.

My sweetheart bent over to draw something from his knapsack. On my bedside table he placed a small box. I gave it a little shake. Ron warned me not to shake it too vigorously.

"Oh, something fragile," I said, as I opened the flaps to lift out the packaging and tissue-covered object. In my hands lay a white ceramic ornament. A knight in armour holding a sword and a shield.

I looked at Ron and back at the soldier. Yes, the two were very alike. Ron always near to help me fight my battles, a warrior standing on guard for me. Strong and noble. Nothing fragile about him.

"My white knight," I said.

"Look a little closer," he said.

What had I missed? Ron leaned over to point it out. "He's wearing a patch over one eye… your warrior is wounded."

He smiled wistfully at me.

I nearly choked. The impact of his message found my self-sorry heart and drew me out of myself. All these times when I feared he had grown indifferent, my warrior was simply finding the best way to manage his own fears. Lost in my own stuff, I failed to see that I was not the only one hurting.

My pain was Ron's sorrow; my broken body was Ron's broken heart. My scars were visible. His were not.

My white knight, my wounded warrior, my treasure. *Lord,* I breathed, *thank You for choosing this honourable man for me. Please help me to be the woman he needs.*

We held hands, soaking up the tenderness of love's promises kept safe with God's help.

~

DAYS 11 to 34

When my kidney began to produce more output, the specialist decided to ease me off dialysis and let the graft do a bit more work. Fewer runs meant more hope. As I began to anticipate the possibility of no longer needing dialysis, joy dared to spring up.

On one of those more hope-filled mornings when Paul wheeled me to the dialysis ward for a shorter run, I imposed on his good will. My longsuffering son endured my commands: plump my pillow, crank up my bed, bring me a drink, hand me my writing bag…

"Anything else, Mom?" he interrupted, his words clipped short.

From my throne I had tossed directives and my loyal servant had quietly served day after day. But clearly he'd had enough.

"Yes," I beamed, "Now, hand me my crown."

Paul stifled a smirk, I giggled, and from the nursing station we heard a few nurses crowing with laughter.

One of them said, "Looks like you are getting better, Liz. We haven't heard a joke from you in ages."

Over the next couple of weeks I was moved to a bright single room in the hostel near the wards, where I could be daily monitored while beginning the transition to self-care. I was even allowed day passes to go out with Ron and the boys for lunch, and take in an evening of jazz with my sweetheart. For our first date since surgery, Ron bought me a gorgeous red print sundress with splashes of yellow.

Finally on a glorious June morning Ron took me home to begin life in a different way. With a functioning kidney and no more dialysis.

~

Three months after my transplant, a beloved friend in Australia called to say she wanted to visit us in Wetaskiwin. Earlier that year her fifty-one-year-old husband Ian — one of Ron's dearest friends – had died in his sleep of a massive heart attack. A young widow at age forty, Karen wanted to reconnect with those who remembered and knew her husband best. We four had been friends and co-workers in our Oakville church two decades earlier and had moved away about the same time. This was our first reunion after all that time.

One late night Karen and I sat in our kitchen talking for hours. The face of my lovely friend was etched with a sorrow I hoped never to experience. She had lost her dearest friend and soul mate without warning. Theirs had been a marriage like ours: two people deeply committed to one another and to the Lord God.

During many tears and cups of tea, we plumbed the depths of her fresh loss.

After a while Karen turned her attention to my pain. She wanted to hear how I had come through it all. Her prayers and letters had followed us through all our years apart. Now she leaned forward to enter as fully as she could into my story.

After reciting some of the highlights in a clinical manner as though they had happened to someone else, I changed focus. I confessed how shocking it felt from my relatively safe vantage point to think about what we had been through. It was hard to grasp how we had survived that. So many trials; so many lonely years for Ron and the boys not having a healthy wife and mom; so many long hours of dialysis and weary strength when I could have done something meaningful with my life.

"All those wasted years," I finished, looking down at my scarred arm.

"Oh no!" my grieving friend protested. "God never wastes our years or our tears."

I could not answer.

She proceeded with care. "Right now, all you can see is waste… but in time we will see more clearly." She paused.

I could hardly see Karen through my stream of tears. How could she say this when her own heart was broken?

"God will show us that He has used every tear for good," she said.

Here was my friend with a heart bathed in one of the greatest sorrows I could imagine, assuring me that neither her tears nor mine were for nothing. They meant something to God. He would redeem them.

"I hope so," I whispered.

~

chapter 12
Sunny outlook, suite escape, ecstatic challenge

I owe much of my recovery to Ron's practical insights and plans to move me forward.

After both our sons moved away from home, we sold our house in Wetaskiwin and bought a condo in Edmonton, close to the University Hospital where my new kidney health could be closely monitored. Meanwhile, Ron commuted back and forth to our hardware business in Wetaskiwin and opened new franchises in Edmonton and Onoway. Ron thrived on multiple challenges.

During my first year with a transplant I experienced a number of serious rejection episodes that threatened the survival of my graft, but all were eventually resolved.

Despite these setbacks we could be found on weekends exploring our new Saskatchewan Drive neighbourhood overlooking the river valley. At first I zoomed along on a three-wheel scooter while Ron tried to keep up. During our scooter walks Ron capitalized on a philosophy he had always believed in — finding the sunny side of things — literally.

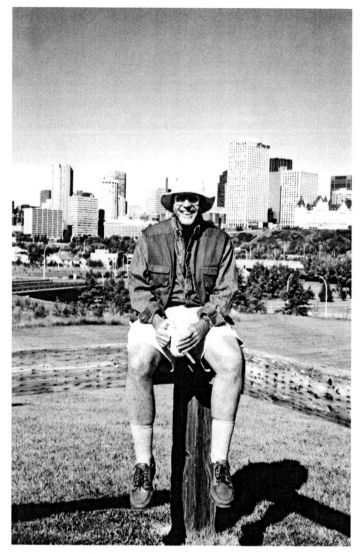

Ron on the sunny side of an Edmonton trail, 1998

Whenever we found ourselves walking in the shadows, Ron pointed out that the other side of the street looked brighter, so we crossed over. If anyone were within hearing distance they might hear us sing, or try to sing, our own off-key version of *The Sunny Side of The Street*. Even when it rained, Ron often remarked, "This isn't the sunny side!" Then breaking out in an imitation of Gene

Kelly dancing in the rain, my crazy man would skip, hop, do a jig, and twirl our umbrella while we both got soaked trying to cross the road. We laughed and kissed, our *Tilley* hats bumping brims. We were surviving the trials and still had much to celebrate.

~

Winter posed another threat for me. During Edmonton's cold icy winters I stayed indoors to avoid falling and breaking my bones, depleted by years of renal failure. This lack of fresh air and exercise affected my morale and strength. As in all matters concerning my well-being, Ron considered how to address this. On several of our visits to Victoria Ron suggested we check out the idea of investing in a tiny suite where I could spend winters and walk outdoors without fear of falling. We targeted a high-rise located in James Bay, close to the waterfront, shopping and bus system.

When the next November rolled around, Ron and I flew to Victoria to settle me into our new cottage in the sky. A few months earlier Ron had gone ahead of me to finalize the purchase and furnish our one-bedroom 680-square-foot suite with the help of Mark and Paul who hauled and arranged the furniture.

As our elevator climbed to the fifteenth story I looked at Ron. I wasn't sure about this choice. Heights were intimidating for me. Holding my hand, my sweetheart led me to the end of the hallway, stopped in front of our door, and turned the key.

Then just like the new husband of thirty years earlier, Ron asked me if he could carry his "bride" over the threshold. He never stopped calling me his bride — and I never tired of hearing it. Sure, I smiled. This was, after all, a new adventure for us — our sweet escape from the harsh realities we had passed through.

With great care Ron lifted me — he needed to watch his bad back — pushed the door open, and carried me into the foyer. Setting me down, he watched as my eyes took in the transformation of the suite into a bright cozy home: a love seat and green leather chairs in the living room, and a new apartment size table and chairs in the kitchen/dining room in forest green and oak. Wall-to-wall windows in every room flooded our tiny place with light and showcased the Victoria Harbour, the Strait of Juan de Fuca and the Olympic Mountains of Washington.

When Ron stepped onto the balcony overlooking downtown Victoria I declined to venture that far. I would cross that threshold another time. Maybe.

I sat down on the love seat and teared up. Ron had lovingly planned this retreat for us, and our sons had been a part of this gift. I was moved. So much tender care in my life.

We spent ten days together enjoying our new home, filling it with bouquets of daisies and carnations chosen by Ron from the outdoor vendor in Cook Street Village. We explored the nooks of James Bay and strolled along the coast of Dallas Road. Well, Ron strolled and I rode alongside on my scooter.

Then the time had come. The part I dreaded.

Ron had to return to his businesses in Alberta. He would be back for a week every month during the winter but I would need to work out how to make the most of my winter weeks alone. I assumed Ron would be so busy he would not miss me as much as I would miss him.

But I often underestimated his feelings for me. Dropping his bags at the door, he turned to give me a farewell embrace before his airport taxi arrived. As we listened to the music playing low on our radio, we found ourselves in a slow dance, holding onto our last few precious moments and the gift that was always our love story.

~

We decided to name our hideaway, *R & L's Suite Escape,* which our talented friend Colleen inscribed in a ceramic plaque for our front door. Loneliness and gratitude for this winter haven drove me to productive use of my time. During my first winter I took exercise classes and short walks around James Bay. I scootered all over town, exploring shops and attending St. Andrew's church up the hill; and in the long dark nights I sat at my typewriter inventing short stories for my correspondence course. The variety of clocks "tocking" back and forth in our apartment not only comforted me but inspired the backdrop for one of my creations. A small Canadian literary magazine, called *Greens*, published this piece of fiction. Ron and I were delighted.

Ron and I talked daily on the phone, keeping one another posted on our daily events. His monthly arrival was always a time of anticipation as I looked for the Airporter to deliver him to our street. Each time he came he noticed how much healthier I looked. On our walks Ron walked alongside my scooter a few blocks and then we traded places. I would poke along with my cane and he would ride my scooter so that I could rebuild the strength in my legs. People passing by often smiled because it seemed odd that I was the one walking when Ron looked perfectly able bodied, which he was. We smiled back, enjoying the joke.

We spent many Christmases in our *Suite Escape*, with our sons joining us for several days.

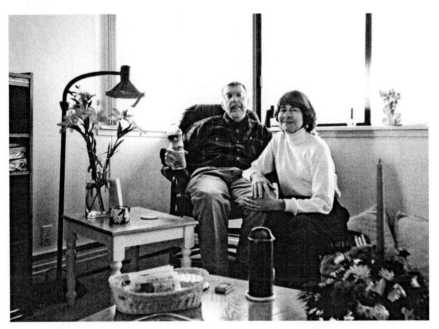

Enjoying renewed health with Ron in our Suite Escape, 1999

Mark ferried over from Vancouver where he worked on films and TV series as a set dresser, lead dresser or electrics. As well, he wrote his own movie scripts as a hobby and possible future career. Paul walked over, since he chose to live in Victoria to study political science and economics at UVic, and ran for their track team. In later years, he took long cramped bus trips from Kamloops where he was completing his bachelor's degree at Thompson Rivers University. When our sons arrived we indulged them with big meals, and listened to their adventures.

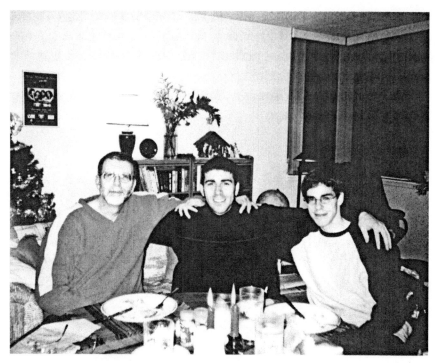

Christmas with my three men, Victoria 2000

~

Every May 1st I began the tradition of sending my brother Dave a card of thanksgiving for his gift of life to me. A few weeks after the third anniversary of my transplant, Dave called Ron. "Is everything okay? I didn't get a card from Liz this year." Ron chuckled and assured Dave I was doing well. "I think Liz is working on something... don't worry, she has not forgotten you."

I certainly had not forgotten. Wishing to thank Dave in a public way, I composed a tribute for him and sent it to *The Globe and Mail*. They hoped to publish it in their essay section before the end of May. My eighty-two-year-old dad, a regular subscriber, knew about the surprise and relished Dave's response. On the day the piece appeared Dad called Dave to stop by his Oakville shop as soon as he could. Apparently my brother's jaw dropped to the floor when he saw the tribute. Later that day, May 30th, Dave called again. "Sis, you're a bit late, but that is some thank you card!" I heard the emotion in his voice. My brother received many phone calls from old friends who recognized him as a hero for giving his sister *A Sacrifice Beyond Compare*.

~

My second Victoria winter Ron persuaded me to take swimming lessons to further strengthen my muscles and endurance. I balked. My swimsuit days were over. And besides, I hated water on my face. Eventually I surrendered my excuses. Hadn't I overcome my fear of heights and ventured onto the balcony these days? Maybe I could overcome this fear as well. A whole lot of praying took place in that pool. After my first class I excitedly announced to Ron that I had done it. "What, did you already learn to swim?" he asked. "No," I laughed, "I showed up." Showing up was half the battle.

The swim sessions were a study in endurance for both my instructor and me. While I often eyed the exit, the young man was gradually inching me toward the deep end. With white knuckles and a yellow heart I gripped the poolside. The day he asked me to get out of the water, I knew this couldn't be good.

It wasn't. When I pulled myself out, dripping and terrified, he said, "Now jump in."

"Does your mother know what you do for a living?" I asked.

When I finally took the leap into water three feet over my head, I came paddling back up, ecstatic with the thrill of challenging danger. No objections when he asked me to jump again and again. I eventually learned to swim like a pro, with my face dipping in and out of the water.

Oh the wonder of overcoming the thing you fear. I had not done it without help from my cheering husband, my instructor and most of all, my God.

~

chapter 13
Suffocating doors, mischievous grin, changing poses

It was while towelling down after one of my swims that I found something unfamiliar. My heart took a plunge. Over my left breast I discovered stony bumps like gravel. Ron insisted I get back to Edmonton for testing. The answer wasn't long in coming. The specialist pulled no punches. "I'm sorry, you have cancer."

Lord, haven't we been through enough trials? What are you trying to do? Ron and I were stunned and heartsick.

I recall standing in church the week before surgery, placing a hand over my chest and whispering to the Lord that I knew He was able to heal me. "But," I added, "If You can bring more glory to Your Name by allowing me to go through this, then I surrender to this."

After I had a radical mastectomy and time of recovery at home, the day arrived to visit the Cross Cancer Center for the verdict on treatment. My new kidney of three years had finally begun to function with efficiency, but now we faced the strong possibility of losing it to chemotherapy and radiation.

Donning a yellow print skirt and yellow sweater set, I decided I might as well face this next step with some flair. Ron and I were ready. The Lord would be with us no matter what. His promise was for always: *I will never leave you nor forsake you.*

It felt suffocating to step through the doors I had passed through many times before, only this time as one of the cancer patients. Quivering under my sunflower bravado, I waited my turn. My name was called. After a consult, I left bewildered.

I had been ready for the fight of my life — but I had been spared. No need for chemo or radiation. No cancer in my lymph nodes. I could walk away.

As I stepped back into the bright Alberta sunshine of that May morning, I said, "Is that all there is to cancer?"

And I began to laugh at the absurdity of my question. I had lost a womanly part of my body to cancer but I did not need to face another mountain at this moment. *Thank you Lord for this reprieve!*

I went home and held up my new red linen dress, the one Ron had chosen for me the week before my cancer surgery. Hanging it in my closet, my wise husband had asked me to savour it until after my surgery and recovery. He understood the healing value of anticipation and hope. That weekend he took me candlelight dining in my red dress of celebration.

Inspired by my husband's loving oversight, I wrote an article featuring our red dress story and sent it to *MAMM* magazine in New York. We were thrilled when they accepted it for publication.

~

During the months that followed surgery I still experienced hills and valleys in learning to adapt to my changed body and the scare of cancer. Ron would often notice my sadness as I undressed for bed. Sometimes he brushed my arm and whispered that I was still beautiful. Other times he urged me to move beyond these scars and not stay stuck in loss.

To express his pride in me, he planned a very special event for me. On one of our date evenings at an Italian restaurant, Ron wore a mischievous grin as he handed me a package and watched me unwrap it. It was a picture frame. Behind the glass I found a note of invitation:

A PHOTO SHOOT HAS BEEN ARRANGED FOR YOU AT THE STUDIO OF DEBBIE BOCCABELLA

You're kidding, my own photo shoot? Ron explained that he wanted a professional photographer to capture the strides I had made to overcome another obstacle to health. One of our jazz friends had recommended Ms. Boccabbella who had done her own recent promo shots.

Debbie made me feel at home when she came to our place to preview my wardrobe and suggest the outfits most camera-friendly: a pair of jeans with a classic white shirt, a little black dress with pearls, and a black sweater and slacks with gold necklace. She recommended I keep my hairstyle natural rather than having it styled at a salon. She would apply my makeup.

The following Wednesday morning Ron dropped me off at the warehouse that housed the photo studio. "Enjoy yourself, my love. Don't worry about how it will turn out." Good advice for a chronic worrier. When I walked into Debbie's studio I found a cloud of white bedding on a big square bed as the set, along with a window draped in filmy white stuff.

I felt like a star, being pampered and dressed and made up and snapped. The photographer told me to keep changing my poses. Standing, sitting, and stretching: some poses with a smile, some with a thoughtful look, and some with laughter. Snap, snap, snap. The morning passed in a happy dream and then it was time to head home.

That evening as I tried to remove my makeup I began to laugh with disgust. The heavy eyeliner smeared, making raccoon eyes that would not wash off; one black blob fell onto my cheek. Ron crept up to the bathroom with his camera, catching me in all my inglorious attire. As he snapped my last photo for the day I stuck out my tongue.

Two weeks later my proofs arrived. I handed them to Ron. Tears filled his eyes as he reviewed the rows and rows of shots. "What?" I asked. "Don't you like them?" When he could speak he replied, "This is how I always see you. Now I hope you can see yourself, too."

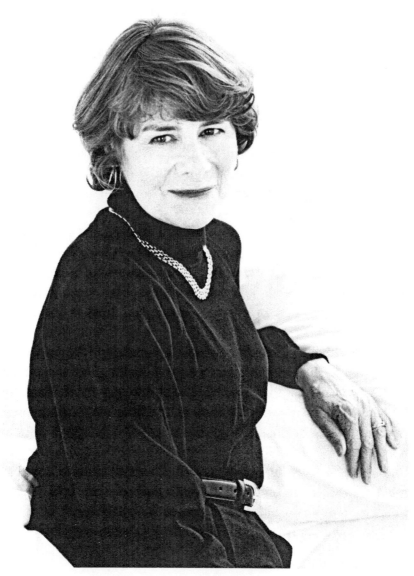

A photo shoot to celebrate cancer recovery, 2000

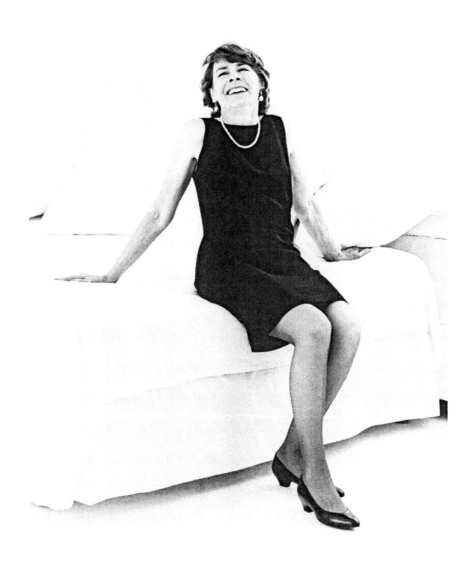

Rejoicing in my return to health

The photographs turned out beyond our best dreams. They were picture perfect. I was delighted that Ron loved them and he was delighted that I was pleased, too.

Since my photos turned out so well, my husband decided it was safe to show me what he had picked up that week. The photo of me in my flannel nightgown with blackened eyes and tongue hanging out! We nearly fell over laughing at the contrast between my before and "after the ball" pictures. Cinderella had lost her slipper and returned home to her broom and ashes. But it had been fun!

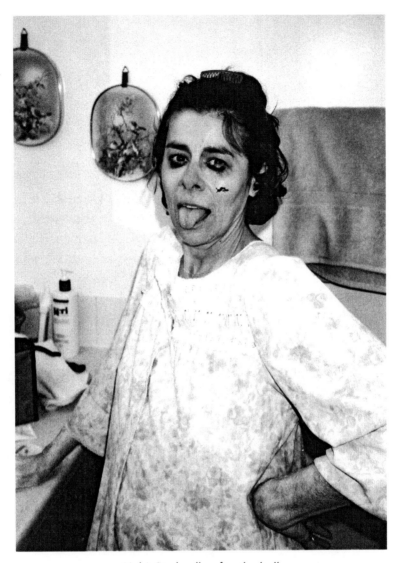

Ugh! Cinderella after the ball

~

reflections

In recent spring times we've been taking an annual road trip through the Rockies in Ron's white '91 Chrysler LeBaron convertible, with top down all the way. A little rain does not deter our enjoyment. The water arcs over us while we stay dry — as long as we don't stop or slow down. Beach towels make handy blotters when we do get caught at a light. As well, we provide plenty of amusement for passing drivers, enjoying the nonsense with us.

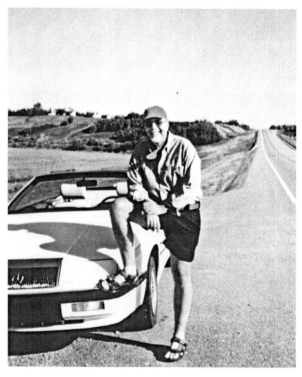

Enjoying the open road with Ron's '91 LeBaron, 2010

This year of 2011 the occasion is our forty-second anniversary.

Dashboard dining saves us time and affords us a moving landscape. Stopping to take out two orders of *Timmy's* breakfast biscuits, we return to our convertible, don our cloth aprons and continue our drive along the Yellowhead Highway, our breath making puffs of fog in the morning chill. I think about how funny we look: Ron with his red apron that happens to match his red ball cap and brown legs in *Tilley* shorts, and I bundled in multi-layers with a blanket and floral apron adding extra layers of warmth.

Before we eat Ron asks me to give thanks for our meal. The thing is he can never hear me because of the wind noise. Though he adjusts his hearing aids he still cannot pick up the sound of my voice. This time I decide to shout "AMEN!" hoping Ron can hear me as well as God can.

Ron grins, "It's a good thing you let me know when you were finished praying — that way I knew when to open my eyes again."

I do a double take and laugh at my husband's teasing.

Ron and I enjoy being together and I am still like a cat in the sun, purring with satisfaction as we share treasured moments together — like meeting for a tea date at a cafe, or holding hands as we take a long stroll to Granville Island from our motel, or spending time with our adult sons who have grown into fine men.

We have much to celebrate. Twelve years have passed since my brush with cancer, our red-dress celebration dinner and my photo shoot. Though it is losing significant efficiency, Dave's kidney is still working for me these fifteen years. None of us dreamed this graft would last so long.

How grateful we feel for having come through miles of adversity with our faith and marriage more durable than ever. As the reader knows by now, the journey has not been an easy ride.

~

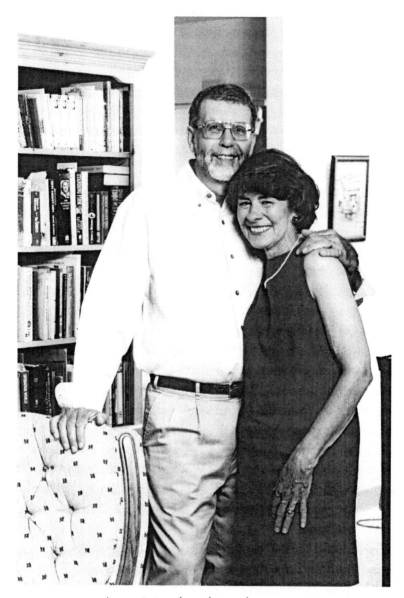

Appreciating the miles we have come

~

Just the way one notices the steep incline one has made upon approaching a hilltop, we get a clearer view of how far we have come by looking back.

Remember the shepherd's pie supper with the enquiring doctor and his wife at the opening of this story? It took place a few years ago and this brings us to the big questions they asked that night about suffering, faith and God.

Let's listen in to part of that conversation…

"Do you think that what you went through made you a better person? Were you angry with God? Bitter? Did your faith in God grow stronger?"

"Marriages often do not survive serious illness. What brought you through?"

"People tell me that there's no point to suffering. They say that nothing good comes from it."

So… is there a point to suffering? Can any good come from it? Does God even care?

With these questions in mind, I have told our story as a way of mining the answers embedded in the scenes.

Looking back, I see that no matter what was happening in our youthful years, our courtship, our marriage, in our years of misdiagnosis, in the Moose Jaw years of dialysis terrors and adjustment, in the transplant process and then cancer, God was present, showing us how to live through it. Our faith in Him did grow and grounded us.

Did our faith falter? Absolutely. Sometimes I felt like throwing in the towel I was so bitter. I often doubted that God cared about us. At times we were too weary to go to church and truthfully answer the myriad questions about my health.

But God proved himself true by giving us room to mourn our losses and even rail at Him. We learned that there is a time to grieve and a time to dance. We realized the healthiness of admitting to ourselves how hard life can get and to grieve our pain as long as necessary.

~

Then came the gentle promptings to move out of the sadness and shadows into a sunnier view of our life. Recall how Ron was always on the lookout for the sunniest side of the street — even in the rain. A change of morale is a miracle not to be taken for granted.

It is true that chronic illness gave us few breaks. Like heat waves rising from the pavement we experienced grief, then relief, then more grief — but hope always reappeared.

God showed us that we don't need to work up joy on our own steam. Rather it is a supernatural result of leaning into Him. As promised in Isaiah 61:3, Jesus gave us "the oil of joy for mourning, the garment of praise for the spirit of heaviness."

~

Now, as we age, new challenges, fears and other emotions take hold. A return to dialysis grows imminent… perhaps another search for a transplant as well. My system carries many rare antibodies that make finding a matched donor a long shot, especially for a senior.

Having traveled the dialysis road before, Ron and I know about the twists and turns. We know it will be difficult to face another series of medical roadblocks but it will be doable. God will help us along the way. He is compassionate and will not waste our tears. He will make our times of trouble count for something good as we learn to depend on Him and not on ourselves.

The Creator of our Universe will go ahead of us. He is not afraid of anything.

We admit the future feels scary for us. Though our circumstances are changing again, God remains consistent. This truth compels us to focus on God's bigger picture — His purpose to redeem us from pointless pursuits and follow Him. Remember that banner of twenty-eight years ago? His message to us remains the same.

Bloom where you are planted, or Bloom where I plant you — at all stages of your life.

Life is about blooming wherever our circumstances take us, by sharing His love and hope with others, and letting His compassion shine through.

Some day Jesus will return for those who hope in Him and what joy there will be when we see His welcoming face — the One who faithfully walks with us all the way to heaven.

"In the world you will have trouble, but let your heart take courage, I have overcome the world." John 16:33

The End

update for 2012
changing circumstances, tricky procedure, unremarkable day

Recently we faced another challenge to my renal health. During a kidney biopsy six years ago, an artery and a vein were mistakenly nicked, resulting in a bulge or fistula where blood began to collect. My specialist hoped it would eventually close over. But it did not do the predictable thing. Instead it gradually grew larger.

Picture a small balloon filling with blood. As it continues to expand it becomes dangerously close to bursting and causing a big mess – and possible loss of the kidney.

To prevent this scenario, a surgeon decided to take the chance of performing a delicate procedure – an angiography — to seal the leak at the neck of the fistula. He warned us it held the risk of significantly reducing or even shutting down my kidney function. Since my function was only at 24% there was not much margin to play with. Yet to do nothing was more risky. I assured this conscientious doctor that many prayers would follow him. He may not have appreciated them but I needed those prayers.

I was quaking in my skin. Lying on that hard table in the chilly procedure room I could not stop trembling. Then a mild sedative was injected into me. Ahhh. Now I was feeling very relaxed without being put out. It was just enough to keep me quiet yet alert.

When the procedure proved to be trickier than expected, the time extended by another hour. The doctor had warned us he might need to stop the procedure if the situation looked too dangerous. He did not know what he would face beforehand because it was unsafe to inject dye contrast to take pre-surgery pictures. Too much dye would compromise my limited kidney function. But pictures were needed.

Only at the exact time of surgery did the surgical team inject dye to see where they were going. The arterial path to the fistula proved to be a gauntlet of loops making it very difficult to thread a wand along this tortuous passageway. Many attempts were made to insert each plug or coil. Meanwhile the patient's body began to shake again.

The doctor asked, "Do you want another shot?" The patient nodded yes. *Send it on down*, I smiled to myself.

Finally the surgeon was able to complete the job. It took five coils to tightly seal the leak. Ron and I are grateful for his attention to detail and determination to perform this procedure. My kidney function dropped to twenty-two percent but has rallied by a few percentage points. Twenty-six percent may not seem like much but it keeps me off dialysis a while longer.

~

When I visited a new family doctor in Victoria this week he reviewed my current renal function and asked how I manage the tension of knowing any day could mean a return to dialysis. I wondered how to answer.

Before I could speak he remarked, "It must be you have faith... in God."

Yes, that is it. Faith in God, no matter what... even in the rain, even in the torrential downpour. Life on the sunny side means carrying an umbrella of trust in the One who is trustworthy above all others.

~

On Fridays Ron and I take a slow stroll from our Victoria apartment into James Bay Village shopping area for our weekly date. First we stop at the Friday thrift store beside James Bay United church to poke around for bargains. Next we browse in the video store for our weekend movies. *Captain America* appeals to the boy in Ron, while a romantic drama set in the twenties draws me in. For some reason Fridays often turn rainy so we look for the sunny side of the situation.

Shall we continue our walk or duck into a coffee shop? *Starbucks* wins. We buy hot drinks and take advantage of their coffee mocha and bakery samples. After reading our newspapers Ron visits the nearby pizzeria and returns with a large slice of mushroom and sausage for us to share. This coffee shop allows all manner of outside food as long as patrons buy something in-store. A cozy way to spend a rainy day.

On our way home Ron carries the umbrella, along with muffins and bundt cake he bought "to use up our ice cream". He said the cake was calling his name. I veer to the right trying to dodge the hydro poles on the narrow sidewalk while Ron tries to keep me dry. We laugh and agree it has been another great date.

~

We are in awe. This Valentine's week I have made it to my 65th birthday. Ron presents me with both *Rogers* and *Callebaut* ginger chocolates. "You won't have to share them," my husband teases since he does not care for ginger. As always he gives me a beautiful *Blue Mountain* card with meaningful words that probably took him an hour to choose. I tear up part way through...

To love you is to not forget the adversity we have overcome, the tears we have shed. Know with clarity and assurance Our Lord will continue to guide us through all future events!

Ron watches me dabbing my eyes. He says, "Thirty years ago the doctor gave you a year. And here you are."

I nod. The miracle is not lost on me.

I want to share this with someone who will appreciate the breadth of the miracle. Dialing the number of the kidney specialist who helped us through the critical Moose Jaw years, I wonder if he will remember us. I hold my breath as his secretary tells him who is on the line.

When "Dr. Rose" answers the phone I ask, "Do you know who this is?"

"Yes, I think so." He sounds tentative.

He considers... throws out some specific details about my case that confirm he has very good recall after three decades. I give him an update; tell him that I spent thirteen years on dialysis and finally received a kidney from a brother that has lasted sixteen years so far.

Dr. Rose is pleased I have taken the time to get in touch. Then he recalls an anecdote that has us both laughing.

"Do you remember when you took me to task for using the term *unremarkable* to describe you in a report?"

"Oh yes I do!" My face reddened. I could not believe he remembered that embarrassing incident.

Unremarkable is a medical term that means the patient's condition has no abnormalities. But I thought he was implying that I was boring and ordinary. I let him know I was not unremarkable.

We laughed at my feisty retort.

When we were done reminiscing I thanked Dr. Rose for helping Ron and myself through a critical time in our lives. He had listened to us and provided sound advice, moral support and humour. He and Jacquie, the social worker, had both been anchors in our storm.

Later in the week a follow-up email arrived from Dr. Rose who could not resist teasing the feisty patient from thirty years before. It read...

I just wanted to thank you again for turning a rather unremarkable day into a great one!

How Ron and I laughed. Life is good and the Giver of life is good to have allowed me to survive these difficult years alongside my amazing husband. With the help of many fine doctors, nurses, family members, friends and acquaintances, what might have been an unremarkable life turned into a truly great one.

"Thanks be to God who gives us the victory in Christ Jesus."
1 Corinthians 15:5

CPSIA information can be obtained at www.ICGtesting.com
Printed in the USA
LVOW08s0255140114

369244LV00001BA/28/P

9 781460 210482